LETTERS
TO
LEIGH

I0127096

By Demonmocker

'One million people commit suicide every year'
The World Health Organization

LETTERS TO LEIGH

All rights reserved, no part of this publication may be reproduced by any means, electronic, mechanical photocopying, documentary, film or in any other format without prior written permission of the publisher.

Published by
Chipmunkapublishing
PO Box 6872
Brentwood
Essex CM13 1ZT
United Kingdom

http://www.chipmunkapublishing.com

Copyright © Demonmocker 2008

Property of Robert Sherman Nix III

Author And Sole owner

LETTERS TO LEIGH

Background

I met love
In the form
Of Leigh
Within
The boundaries
Of a hospital
Established for
The treatment of
Persons who happen
To have illness,
That is,
We are people
Who do have
A brain structure.
With a slight difference from yours.
Just as whomever you see, hear, touch, smell, and
Speak with are slightly, at least, different
From yourself or anyone else on this earth, ever.

Yet love is what we extend for we find that we have
An abundance that we freely afford to you
While we ask for little from your love in return.

Love, kindness, joy
The healing from within That may pass from person to person.

Leigh and I met in April 1996 then parted in May.

LETTERS TO LEIGH

The original poems herein reconstructed
Were written in May 1996 to august 1996.
In September of 1996,
I did receive electroconvulsive therapy
For the untranslatable pain of depression resulting
from finding myself
Deep within a loss of hope for a love felt by myself
that I had not ever
 fully come to have known, for she may have been
for my future a lifetime of love.
To that point in my life, the final addition of a loss
for a love that was tragically somewhat
understandable and somewhat not,
Added upon a needless loss of my trade involving
the needless loss of my friends after the needless
loss of the prospects of an equal education
After loss upon loss with losses in between losses
which did lead to the losses and eventual gains of
my spirit and mind,
Perhaps involving the working out of something
better for me.

I have visited hospitals seven times since the loss
of my trade,
Three since the last time that I saw Leigh.
At times my mind is a medley of emotions yet I
think, yet I feel,
Yet I retain the place within that is called upon to
write
That she helped to lead me into and bring from
within my self.

Page xxx and page xxx

LETTERS TO LEIGH

Were written in 2005
And page xxx
Was written in 2006.

I may have to thank many people for helping me
to be able
To accomplish this body of poems, which I hope to
have rewritten
In a manner that is correct for the better refection
on the mentally ill
Who are often thought to be incorrect.
Although are we all as men and women either
correct or incorrect.
If I am incorrect then I am correctable.
Open your eyes to our difficulty and unstop your
ears to our reason.

The disabled are not by definition to be considered
incapacitated.
We retain a wholesome mind.

The disabled are not by definition incapacitated.
We are disabled enough to meet the guidelines
Of the U.S. social security administrations
requirements
In regard to being eligible to receive disability
benefits.
Thereafter we find the term disabled often in the
common use of many who would help us and
some who would take advantage of us.

LETTERS TO LEIGH

Within our inner selves there are parts that must
not ever become disabled.
many of us feel pain more intensely and love more
abundantly, do not allow us to become lost.

If you know someone in adequate care who is in
some need
Anyone may visit on or call any attorneys office
For a list of toll free telephone numbers
Of attorneys in your state.
If you are unable to acquire the services of an
attorney,
Ask for a list of mental health advocacy
Organizations in your state.
No one is disabled in the purpose of life
For we all do have abilities

The U.S. government is not known to pay benefits
To persons of shadow or ghost-people.
Please do not allow your loved one to become as
such.
Pray with us.

LETTERS TO LEIGH

Indebtication

The nourishment of the emotions
Include love, kindness, and joy.
Such is what saved me from
The pool of oblivion.

The pool

I found myself lost
In the pool
Of oblivion
And was alone
Except for silent
Jesus Christ
My lifeguard
As his angels
Were all
Around me
From being scooped
From the bed
Into the wheelchair
As my head
Did nod
And was pushed
Down halls
Into an elevator
To the basement
For the treatment
Five times
Was it good for my mind
Was it to erase
Leigh from my hearts place

LETTERS TO LEIGH

It didn't help
Because there her I have kept.

The author.

Letters to Leigh

By:

Demonmocker

Robert Sherman Nix iii.

LETTERS TO LEIGH

For true royalty

Also

To the heroes of mental health;
Whether within or without

The simple tale from a mind that was lost then
found
Of a love that was found then lost
And of a soul though lost yet found.

The author.

God is my ally

LETTERS TO LEIGH

LETTERS TO LEIGH

Table of contents

LETTERS TO LEIGH

32   To face joy or sorrow
33   For me to enter through the door
34   Please save the sad song
35   Your memory
36   After awhile
37   Dream emergency
38   I tell you now
39   Hoping that soon
40   Let us keep all of that
41   Love loves love
42   Your taste
43   And help myself to love
44   I shall be loving you
45   To begin a love letter
46   By my soul fed
47   For just a few moments more
48   As long as we are together
49   Myself alone
50   Happy you should be
51   We may mend our sweet sorrow
52   I am still not believing
53   Before we part
54   You turned with that stare
55   Mine own that was not ever left behind
56   I look into your eyes
57   I shall be in preparation
58   She has my heart
59   Do anything for you that i could
60   I miss you now as then
61   Everywhere that i go
62   How deep my love does go
63   Just hold me
64   Of the broken heart that we had

LETTERS TO LEIGH

65   Like an ocean at low tide
66   Love that will stay
67   I know that you love me true
68   Is your heart to haunt?
69   Just hold me close and near
70   To make you my own
71   All of my thoughts are safe with you
72   There are thoughts hidden
73   Yet when we meet then
74   I will take your hand in mine again
75   Anytime day or night
76   Love that waits upon a rainy day
77   If only I may be your friend
78   The wind and the rain
79   Yet the silence does fill my ears
80   Only time may tell
81   An emotional healing
82   As I love you tenderly and dear
83   Love is only one step away
84   True love is not ever wrong
85   When I have part of you to feel
86   Then unto me you may give your deepest
emotion
87   A loving fool
88   I love you Leigh
89   Where cupids arrow aimed
90   Tis love at first sight
91   You know me Leigh
92   Yet when I am all alone
93   From me into your heart to stay
94   Around my heart
95   Of from where love pours
96   The sounds of our heart are forever sealed

LETTERS TO LEIGH

97   Must be that I shall not ever erase
98   May be that one day I shall be whole
99   To you little dove
100   Drinking in loves wine
101   For who may escape the power of love
102   Go ahead, give it some thought
103   Amixing lonely ink with tears
104   You are still knocking on my loves doors
105   What do I do now?
106   Love is knocking at the door
107   Then her smile
108   Loves seeds have been sown
109   We hold our love in our hands
110   I love you Leigh, I am for real
111   I want you to know that I am waiting
112   All in due time
113   I shall find you one day
114   Sometimes I think that I am losing
115   Into loves sweet hell
116   Sometimes I think that I am losing
117   My heart is on the pyre
118   When we are home
119   I am going to sound loves bugle call
120   To leave you with a tear stain in your eye
121   By your own choice
122   Yet my favourite way
123   Watching the wind blow
124   Then we will have not more good-byes
125   Do you think, after all?
126   Just take me back to then
127   Love together we will share
128   Love to make your heart mend
129   Let love come to the fore

LETTERS TO LEIGH

130   Inside of your heart
131   Let us live again
132   Whisper sweet words into your ear
133   You I love so much
134   When we feel loves dart
135   That you might so live
136   Hoping that love will start
137   When you are all alone
138   There I shall stay
139   Like a nest
140   We may spread our love around
141   Would you care for more?
142   To make you whole
143   Let us let love be
144   You say, be a friend
145   So that your love is bare
146   Softly, I have a friend
147   I will bring you joy
148   Have not fear
149   If I only had the treasure
150   Love is not fair
151   Until I feel
152   Like fine wine
153   Around my heart
154   Will I maintain faith?
155   You will not lay me down
156   shall we not have a choice
157   That all of your love is not showing
158   We must make two, one heart
159   Then from there take a sip
160   My soul it is that you soothe
161   Having not spite, nor hate
162   From the heart

LETTERS TO LEIGH

163 Down to the end
164 Like a sweet tart
165 Always nice to me
166 Begging you to bring your tear
167 About my hearts incision
168 From my soap bubble
169 Always doing something good
170 Trying to not do anything wrong
199 Deep down inside
200 That would be a small price to pay
201 Underneath loves fount
202 Whatever you do, wherever you are
203 I am dying a death that is soft
204 I am living not a fable
205 In my need
206 My love did bloom
207 Am I not down on my knee
208 Could it be that you are the woman of my life
209 For when you love somebody
210 I do love my love fount
211 Yet one heart
212 You are still my hope so fond
213 I shall someday be holding you
214 I should not find love a chore
215 All love without pride
216 I will take my time
217 To hold near
218 Yet I never know
219 My torment
220 Love is what I am talking about
221 I am showing you all of my feeling
222 My heart as of yet does remain tore

223 To forever, as time has the sand
224 When there are more than one sweet rose
225 Because my love is deep
226 I have said it many times
227 A new love flow
228 Now I have my heart open
229 When I ever think of you
230 Another day
231 I never meant for you any harm
232 I began with only half of a chance
233 An emotional healing
234 Something I measure others upon
235 The first stone has been cast
236 You may do to me not a greater wrong
237 Back again into my arms
238 I wonder how many words there are left
239 For she has made it known
240 By love you are surrounded
241 I am waiting on my woman
242 Then out of all the confusion
243 Only for you I do concentrate
244 One day we shall drink a toast
245 If only my wife you were to be made
246 To find that nothing has changed
247 I now raise my bid
248 Because the love does flow on
249 Because love is to be found there
250 Never the fool
251 More love letters to thee
252 This too is how I feel
253 Being careful not to fall
254 I am calling day and night
255 If you are sad

256 I cannot be caught
257 I need to hear your voice
258 For I have to say
259 To prevent a tear
260 I have need to call
261 My love is as strong
262 Out of reach like a dove
263 When I am so far away
264 To a cherished place
265 For the love that I hold
266 We feel bold
267 I just have to see
268 Yet your love was laying there
269 Of you I thought
270 To build into her a flame
271 On making it into heaven
272 Some peace of mind
273 Waiting to be felled
274 Yet you do still hold sway
275 For love has not forsook
276 To be cheerful
277 Near or far away
278 Your hearts tender fruit
279 Learn to love again
280 That does never leave me all alone
281 In finding you
282 The many ways
283 To follow the flame
284 Even if there is not a song
285 Upon loves good fruit
286 As I go through life
287 Holding her by her glove
288 You want to put the fire out

LETTERS TO LEIGH

289   My heart yet demanding
290   Down my love do I lay
291   Onto loves garden
292   If that is to be
293   A love dew delicious
294   In my hand until warm
295   A special situation
296   All here safe and sound
297   Then love moved into my vein
298   Dare you to enter glory's portal
299   Waiting, waiting to catch her eye
300   With the words that I have woven
301   Into loves cup
302   I am always asking
303   I wanted to help her out
304   I received that love for free
305   When upon me you shed loves dew
306   Feel free to take my love
307   The same in fears
308   Just me and you
309   Into love that is true
310   After I give unto you a gentle shove
311   These thoughts of love I am thinking
312   Please do not feel bad
313   I am a friend that is true
314   If you cannot see
315   A way to stay in love
316   While I stood ready for her call
317   Loves loosening coil
318   Loving everything
319   New red shoes
320   It is never too late
321   Take, hold, give

LETTERS TO LEIGH

LETTERS TO LEIGH

LETTERS TO LEIGH

Twenty-eight years of broken mirrors

I have broken mirrors, three or four
As a child I have broken, busted, and tore
So my bad luck did accumulate
Then in my teenage years these traits
Only brought in my class
From up in front, back to last
All of my friends were best friends though
Some thought I was just a delinquent, yet not slow
I gave my all to my best friends
This seems to still be my trend
Then all of my friends say that I did to them wrong
Still I played for them wine and song
Until to me all of my friends went past
I stopped and looked behind me at last
There was someone waiting
For me to turn and greet him
I did not trip, I did not fall

LETTERS TO LEIGH

Twenty-eight years of broken mirrors cont.

Because Jesus took me in and I shall
Have not a regret nor forsake him
His words are tender, his load is light
He does stay with me through the night
When I am in need of my best friendly
I turn around and he is there to hold me
Do not ever think that there is not a God
The people who know will all nod
For the precious son is the friend that is best
He does not ask for silly test
If you need a friend that will last and last
You all may be a friend of Jesus Christ
Once when all of my friends had left me
Only Jesus was left so I took him
Now as he ever does walk beside of me, we
Together keep my bad luck trim.
Amen

So let us stay in love

I am surrounded by strangers in this place
I know that you are too
No one here may know me, they just smile at my
face
They think that they know
You, tho no one may know you
As you do
No one may know me so
Let us stay in love
Like a pair of gloves
We shall fit together
No one will ever sever
We will walk hand in hand
Toward the Promised Land
Where will near be a tear
For no one will know fear
No one to run away from
Only peace and joy within our home
With little children running round
Listening to their sweet, sweet sound
So let us stay in love
For we are surrounded by strangers,
Fear and anger
So let us stay in love.

LETTERS TO LEIGH

All of those prayers did not go to waste

All of those prayers did not go to waste
During those sleepless nights
I was not awoken in vain
By all the sweet kisses that I may still taste
Yet being sleepless gave way to morning light
All of those prayers did help ease the pain
Now I lie like baby soft
Like a mouse up in the loft
Because I know that you love me so
I close my eyes then asleep I go.

When next we meet

When next we meet
All sorrow will be made sweet
When next we speak
Love from our one heart shall leak
When next we look
Our hands will have shook
When next we touch
We shall feel our love
When next we kiss
We will feel sweet bliss
When next we meet
Sweet love we shall greet.

LETTERS TO LEIGH

Facing the fortnight

Fourteen days until I see you
Now listen for all of my words are true
Only an hour past I took your hug
Was my blood pounding, was my heart tugged
Thirteen days until I see you
I have unpacked my shirts and shoes
Twelve days until we next touch
I am laying heartsick on the couch
The days until we meet number eleven
You are helping me to find my heaven
Now the days number ten
My love for you is strong my friend
We are now down to number nine
I write a letter line after line
The days that are left total eight
Please do not let this letter be too late

Facing the fortnight cont.

We are now standing before seven
I am now walking downhill toward my heaven
Last count of days came to be six
Lord, my love for Leigh I shall not mix
On the afternoon of the fifth
I hope that I will make your spirits lift
On the fourth I am hoping
As I am wondering how you are coping
Only two days left
Our feeling and love I still felt
Now we have one day more
Then our heart shall feel love galore
(p.s. I noticed that I skipped the third day,
I will just leave it that way).

LETTERS TO LEIGH

Yet the pleasure is mine

There is something that I have been
Meaning to ask, friend,
When you poem poetry
Do you feel something like glory
Does it make you feel
That with Gods approval you have been sealed
Or does the feeling make
You feel fine to create
Hoping to invite others to participate
I cannot remember which
Of us pulled our poetry switch
All I know...
Is that I hear yours and wow!
We can each enjoin
With each others poem
Yet the pleasure
Of writing is light of measure
Because in reading yours I do find pureness
While sometimes mine are just a mess
So between us as to whose is fair
I think you will agree that mine cannot compare.

LETTERS TO LEIGH

The girl with the light brown hair

Lord, we are just friends now
Me, and the girl with the light brown hair
Lord, you chose her name to be Leigh
Yet you did not choose her for me
Lord, I am not angry, I am not mad
For I know that you do not do anything for bad
You are full of wisdom, full of grace
I have a heart of leather, brain of lace
I do not know for us what is best
In this game of life and great love quest
Yet if it is possible in your grand design
I would love for us to be together for all time
 If that is not to be
I shall still love her through eternity
When that eternity is all done
Maybe I will be ready for you then to take me
home
When we get there
I shall wash your feet with my tears
Then dry them with my hair
I will ask you and pray
(While I am there)
Lord in the new day
Please bring to heaven the girl with the light brown
hair.

LETTERS TO LEIGH

No one may make my love to go away

No one may take
This necklace away
No one may make
My love to go away
No one may replace
This ol love necklace
No one may send
Me to another friend
No one may ask
Me to do such a task
No one may look at my face
To see where I have wiped tears away
No one may take this necklace away

No one may make my love to go away cont.

Yet some one could say
Being friends with you I will never lay
Down, no not until the last day
Some one could tell
Me truly how they feel
Some one could give me a hug
For then these sad feelings I could shrug
Some one could give me a kiss and laugh
That I may hide my joy behind a cough
Yet being no one as I am
I shall sit and take it as a lamb
From start to finish
First to last
I have placed my bets
All of my love cash
However it does go
Be it so
Because this is true:
No one may make
My love to go away.

The only thing missing

Being married to me
Is going to be as a fantasy
Life will be a delight
Inside of my paradise
No fretting, no fussing
Nor fighting, nor cussing
I shall lay myself down
She will caress my crown
Then as I escort her around town
She will never see me frown
When from there we get back
I shall use all of my tact
To keep her in the mood
For to her I shall woo
All of my deep emotion
Until her ego is well lotioned
We shall have all of this fun
In then out of the sun
From dawn
Until her love is daily won
All of this we will have
Also true love
The only thing missing
Is the name of
The girl
That I will be kissing.

LETTERS TO LEIGH

The feeling is not missing

I am wishing that I could write
To you a new poem type
Not the kind of true love
For we have given that a gentle shove
While it is not too late
For us to appreciate,
I am trying to find
In my mind
Words that are chaste
Tho pleasant to taste
For me to begin
To love you as a friend
The feeling is not missing
In this word listing
It is just that as a friend
My mind will not listen
It still does want to write
The old poem type
Yet I am learning
While my mind is yearning
To communicate
(even tho it is now late)
It is still going strong
In the way that is wrong
Yet together
We shall tether
Each other
For we are ever sister and brother.

LETTERS TO LEIGH

I will kiss her ring again

I met a ding a ling
I said I shall kiss her ring
I met a ding a ling
I said I shall kiss her ring
I became her escort
I kissed her ring again
Then to her I paid court
I kissed her ring again
In then out of doors
I kissed her ring again
When she wept, when it poured
I kissed her ring again
Going in then coming forth
I kissed her ring again
Till one day, I headed north
I kissed her ring again
She wrote me happy letters
I kissed her ring again
When she called, it was still better
I kissed her ring again

I will kiss her ring again cont.

As she went home with her ex-husband
I kissed her ring again
I met a ding a ling
I said I shall kiss her ring
Now I am a ding a ling
Yet who will kiss my ring.

LETTERS TO LEIGH

It is almost Easter

Sitting in this empty room
All dark and lonely gloom
Carpet wall to wall
With two windows, that is all
There is for the sun
This decor is not fun
Wallpaper throughout the same
Some flowers, although I do not know the name
There is a bulletin board
With pictures of people who have been here
before
There are two dining room tables
While outside there is an old horse stable
There is a desk and a chair
For the staff to watch us in our lair
There is a filing cabinet
Our meds are locked up in it
Against the other wall sits its twin
For them to keep our checks in
All in all, it is a dreary place
Both dungeon rack and mace
To all of us poor unfortunates
Who have been stuck in a place-like-this
It is almost Easter
Yet we sit and fester
In this place commonly known
As the mental health group home.

LETTERS TO LEIGH

Then with my heart coping

I shall be home soon
Going or coming, one
Or the other, maybe
I shall not ever leave
I will just wait by the phone
Perhaps to keep check on the dial tone
Waiting and hoping
Then with my heart coping
Wishing that there was a call
To me from you above all
I shall not be coming home late
Then find that it is my fate
Your call to have missed
When you might have needed me most
Maybe you are out in the rain
Is your heart in pain?
Could you just want to say hello
Should you remember that I am a good fellow
that I am not the type
To mess up your life
Yet that I am a friend
Before all remember
That I am here to rend
To you comfort and cheer
I shall soon be home
I will just wait by the phone.

LETTERS TO LEIGH

Yet the fact of the matter

Let us just pretend
(For a little while) ac
That we had never become friends
I would have not known your style
You would not have shown to me the color of your eyes
I would not have heard your talk
Nor kept up with your walk
Together we would not have spent
Our dollars and our cents
Then shared a candy bar
While we talked about your car
I would not have had a haircut
Nor have noticed the shape of your butt
When you met me you said hey man
While I thought that you were a fine woman
Just please do not treat me as a mister
Because you are forever more to me than a sister
Yet the fact of the matter
Is that blood is thicker than water
As it so should be
Tho being a friend is free
As the air that we breathe
Now as we add up the cost
Of what we have lost
We shall find it to be quite small
Because now we are friends, that is all.

LETTERS TO LEIGH

The blow that fell

 I am going back to him said you
I have heard the wind blow too
I still love him, it is true
I have heard the wind blow too
This time I know that he shall do
I have heard the wind blow too
The spirit he has is like new
I have heard the wind blow too
Now he does want little baby blue
I have heard the wind blow too
He shall not become mad then kick his shoes
I have heard the wind blow too
All of his bad ways have just flew
I have heard the wind blow too
We shall make our old life new
I have heard the wind blow too
I know a girl just for you
I have heard the wind blow too
Her years older than me are two
I have heard the wind blow too
Your happiness shall be perfect, just her and you
I have heard the wind blow too
I said I shall give it time, you are yet only twenty-
two
Now she has heard the wind blow too.

LETTERS TO LEIGH

Yet for you

This cigarette smoking
Just is not joking
Like it used to
Yet for you
Let me be concerned
(I do not intend toward you any harm)
May my manners be undone,
Even if I am wrong
You have your life
Before you as a wife
Then mother
Twice over
Yet if you are addicted
Like me you are not licked
For there is always hope
That we may come off of this dope
Just cut your smoking in half
How ever many packs
The progress you make
Will only take
That truly active life
Far from disease and strife
Then you must also remember this
Ol lady kind
It will help to keep your body members
Refined.

LETTERS TO LEIGH

Just look at me

Some like it sweet and black
While taken in a Cadillac
Some like it with sugar and crème
Wide at both ends, thin in between
Some like the fancy stuff
Soft outside yet inside rough
Some like that-that is instantly ready
Fix it as you please, Joe or Freddy
Some like it handed from my sister
Do not tell where you found it, mister
Although for myself
I do not want any off of the shelf
I have never been too particular
As long as it is not bitter
I will take mine black
I shall take mine plain
I will take mine sweet
I shall take mine creamed
Good is good
It is all the same
Although if I must whisper
Which I prefer
Just look at me
Then you may see
That I would love to have you up
 Giving to me my cup.

LETTERS TO LEIGH

Yet please do not worry

I am trying to write a letter
To help you feel better
Stuck how I know you are
Not allowed even the use of your car
An innocent victim
Of the mental health system
They feed to you dogs tired meat
While you do crave grapes and sweets
Shower this morning, shower today
You are not dirty tho you cannot wash it away
The staff wakes you up
Yet you are still sleepy
Did you pull out your cup
Then in it did pee-pee
Soon off to breakfast you go
One sock and two shoes
 then what do you then have
Only soybean on a slab
When you are done with that poor joke
You go on out to smoke
Then all of the bums come on
To gnaw your kindest of bones
Yet please do not worry
Or feel contrary
Because from home to there
It is from there to back home.

LETTERS TO LEIGH

Like everyone else

I cannot answer for you
Yet for me this is true
This writing attraction
Is quite fascinating
I find myself taming
These words that I have been naming
 I am not sure quite how
When I cannot name myself now
I cannot tell where this has came from
It may have came from my home
As now I sit here chewing gum
To keep my brain from growing numb
Then rearrange my glasses
Hoping to prepare this paper for the masses
I wonder,
Then ponder
Just how do you feel
When you are on a spill
Of words and thoughts
oughts and noughts
this and that
Pulled out of your hat
Do you find
That it s good for the mind
Or have you just felt
Like everyone else.

LETTERS TO LEIGH

Somehow, I know,

Would it have been so bad
If I had
Not written you such long winded
Letters, would you have minded
If we had never met
Then I had not
Given you a ring set
In love
Would you have minded,
Little dove
Somehow, I know,
Although now it does not show
Me you would have missed
If me you had not had to kiss
Whose hand would you say that you did hold
When you so felt bold
If you had to do it all over again
Who would have been your friend
Now, I hope that you do not mind
Because I know that you are kind
If it is not too late
For me to participate
I would like to attend
On you as a friend
 if that should seem for you to be right
I shall take your sister
While I weep into the night.

.

Thou must be kind

I cannot just walk away
Without having something to say
I cannot just turn my face
Without some saving grace
I cannot just turn my back
Then leave my sack
Of dreams behind
Thou must be kind
To me right now
Because I do not know how
To put my thoughts
Where they would have fought
Or if my words could
Speak as they should,
Also, my hands are all wrong
Like they do not quite know where they do belong
All of the body language
Is sending the message
That I do not know
What to say or do
Thy pity I may deserve
Yet thy mercy I would love
Thou has placed me here
On the verge of tears
Just remember that it is his fashion
Always for us to show compassion.

LETTERS TO LEIGH

Beginning with the first Easter day

There is a bird singing
If anyone is up to playing
There are daffodils
If anyone would like to feel
There are winters old leaves
To crunch underneath
There are old trees
Sycamore and hickory
There is some fresh green grass
With dew-drops shining like glass
There are some prickly shrub
Just mind how you do rub
There is a garden of flowers
Where the rose bushes tower
There is pine bark and mulch
Please feel free to touch
There are ants of different sizes
Hurrying home with their prizes
There is concrete for walking
With chairs for talking
The sun is up and shining
So the children are not whining
Let us please leave the hateful
Then show that we are thankful
For the promises that were made
Beginning with the first Easter day.
Amen.

LETTERS TO LEIGH

We do feel one another's heart breaking

Make faces for me
For all of my own,
I said then she
Poked her tongue out at me
Make a funny face
Use your glove of lace
Play peek-a-boo
While I tie her highness shoe
Make faces for me
Especially today
I will take snap-shots
Of your silly spots
To me they shall be dear
As I hold them near
 I shall have a display
Of how you look today
Please, use your facial art
 try to play your part
Just look at me,
Smile and say cheese
You I will keep catching
When you think that I am not watching
 yet the one that I shall love most of all
Is where you cry and bawl
For with each picture that I am taking
We do feel one another's heart breaking.

LETTERS TO LEIGH

Yet what about the father

Have you ever stopped and thought
While you pulled your socks off
How it would feel
To have your feet nailed
Then be hung upon a cross
Or what if he was your son,
A lone and only one,
What if this young one
(Who without knowing sin)
For that you may atone;
Became yours and your friends
Then you should walk to heaven
Where you may come in
Yet what about the father
How he must have felt
As they struck Jesus
Then left angry welts
Tho that was his plan
To save man
From Satan's idees
That we do as we please
his son to have lost
Was what it cost
He was hung on the tree
To save us, his family
God loves us that much.
Amen.

LETTERS TO LEIGH

I shall not play

I am hoping that I find you
Before this letter is due
You are who I am looking
For
 I am knocking
At the door
I have come a long
Way
I cannot be wrong
I shall not play
You are calling
Me today
I am falling
For you in that way
We shall play and laugh
Until
We cough
Then stand still
As we feel
Friendship
Soften
Like cotton
It
May
Not happen
To
All of us that often.

LETTERS TO LEIGH

Like a waterfall

The sun is setting
On my dream
I am not fretting
I have kept the fight clean,
Now I have a choice
Either to make a sad noise
Or to rejoice
Then let love
Take its course
Turning and twisting
Spraying and misting
With a gurgling call
Like a waterfall
Already set
For getting us wet
Yet only cool heads
Are meant for the rapids
So dreams and setting suns
Go and they come
Then it is never easy
To face reality
Yet my reality, I fear
Shall bring me a tear
For now there is a full moon,
While the sun is setting
Before my dawn.

LETTERS TO LEIGH

From my first step I did never look back

I left today at 8:10
Reaching for the wide open
Spaces
I left knowing
That I would not leave any traces
With a spring in my step
I covered landmarks and spaces
I walked quietly
I prayed silently
I could not buy a coke
Only had I five smokes
I passed by my sisters workplace
I never needed to tie my laces
When I was half-way there
I breathed the fresh air
I combed my hair in the wind
Then waved at a passing friend
I put a smoke to my lip
With my comb on my hip
 I passed the city sign
My feet began to whine
 I walked faster
Until the sign I-went-past-her
Then what did my eyes greet,
Mama, driving in sleet
From my first step I did not ever look back.

LETTERS TO LEIGH

To face joy or sorrow

Now I am in a worry
I hope not to be sorry
About what may happen tomorrow
Shall it bring sorrow?
Will thy tears follow?
I must admit
I am almost relieved that you was not
There
When I called from here
Yet I have not fear
I will not let it near
There is nothing to be afraid of
When, as I am, you may be softly tough
With I want to say full
Of feelings so dull
That it will take me some
Time to leave you alone
Time is what I won
Today as I call for you on the phone
Tho I shall be true
As to what I must do
I must follow through
With coming tomorrow
To face joy or sorrow
I shall still be ahead
For my brain is of lead.

LETTERS TO LEIGH

For me to enter through the door

Now I am home
The radio is on
The kids are in bed
Bathed and fed
Mama is lying on the couch
Breathing as a feathers touch
Little things upon the shelf
I check the oven...nothing is left
Little puppy at the door
Leaving tracks across the floor
Old tom-cat all curled up
Has his paw inside of his cup
Old heater has the pilot light on
Ready to go, yet now turned down
All of the lights are turned down low
Now the fridge should not make the fuse blow
Dishes draining in the sink
Faded roses make the link
On the table top
Broom and mop
Put up for the night
Back door closed nice and tight
I am sitting here in this chair
Playing idly with my hair
All this has waited and much more
For me to enter through the door.

LETTERS TO LEIGH

Please save the sad song

If you have to tell
Me something that is sad
Please do not get mad
If I have taken all that I had
Just to help gently place it into thy head
Not to shoot me down dead
While my emotions bleed red
Until I have fed
My love reservoir
Before au revoir
Just come out and smile
Please take a sweet while
Before my soul you tear
Through my numb ears
As all of my male merit
You flail within the spirit
My heart please do not take
Then any harder make
My shoulders may slump
More as the closer you approach to the hump
While with a sad face
 A tear begins to slowly downward trace
I will not be there long
Please save the sad song
All this as I near
Adding silent prayer.

LETTERS TO LEIGH

Your memory

I am going to be careful
With my fist full
Of photos
Even the so-sos
Because all will be
Your memory
Ready
For me
If I feel bold
Then need to hold
Those
Close
I may grin
Yet not lend
Twould be a sin
Because I must win
For my friend
Poems to send
To let her know
For me to show
That she is not losing
She is creating from her posing
Then from her inspiration
Added to my perspiration
From these photos
The beauty will grow.

LETTERS TO LEIGH

After awhile

No one may say that they caught
You with a fault
From the tip of your toe
To the top of your do
I know you will not slip
Then come to accept
Any sad poems that I try,
Any one that would make yourself cry
Because I do not want
For you to vaunt
That weapon
Against my plume
I shall not try
To make you cry
I only for you care
While I wish that you would share
Feeling some ecstasy
With my word-play
 if that is a sin
I shall take my pen
Then lend
All of my mind
Toward making you grin
For I will win
After awhile
From you a smile.

Dream emergency

Good night
Please let
The sweet dreams
Please do not
Bite
Be
Alarmed
The
Pleasure
You just
Felt
Is only
A test
In the
Event of
A real
Dream
That bite
You just
Felt
Would have
Been followed
By a broadcast
On your
Dream emergency
Station
I repeat
This is only a test.

LETTERS TO LEIGH

I tell you now

You probably know
By now
That when I write
I do so in a way that is private
You probably cannot tell
That which I have kept hidden so well
I tell you now
That I am not exactly alone
Before I am done
For over time and space
I happen to see your face
Then I bring your hands
To help move my pen
Before I am done
I bring the rest of you on
Until I have you all alone
I ask
Then you help me with my task
There is nothing wrong
With this kind of song
I feel
A special
Soothing thrill
Because no one
May ignore your body
As they gently take your spirit
Then cuddle it
Like me.

LETTERS TO LEIGH

Hoping that soon

They may think that they will keep us apart
As sweethearts
Do they think that they will win?
To them I only bend
For I will not break
Or take
Their unspoken words
Into me as swords
I shall use as my shield
Thoughts of you child
While this battle
Rages on I will put a saddle
Up on my songs
Through the air shall I then roam?
Through dark forest and darker gloom
Risking untimely death and certain doom
Hoping that soon
Fate will grant me a boon
To make my journey short
That I will soon arrive at your port
Where I shall give out a great shout
Then look all about
Out you will come
To welcome me home
Coming near to make it quite clear
That you were perfectly near
Forever to myself more dear than dear
If only I had in my minds eye peered.

LETTERS TO LEIGH

Let us keep all of that

I am going to find Leigh
One day
She is far away,
I will not find her today,
I must stay
Home
Near the phone
To answer a ring
With a ring of my own
To hear her pleasant sound
Coming along
Is going to be so sweet
I shall ask her to repeat
I am going to find her
One day
 I shall ask her to share
One home to stay
In
Then play
To win
Real love
From above
Heaven sent
Into our tent
Let us keep all of that
Under our hats
Let it always remind me
That I am going to find Leigh.

Love loves love

Maybe a year
From today
This tear
Will trade
Itself for a grin
With my laugh joining in
Maybe then
After now has been
I shall run this frown
Right out of town
My joy shall bloom
Until there is not room
On this earth
For less than mirth
Love loves love
For it does not ever rove
All around
Over town
Love quietly waits
Holds open the gate
Waiting for loved ones
To come on home
In that way
I will wait a year
Then a day
Before the next tear
Does find the way
To there forever stay.

LETTERS TO LEIGH

Your taste

I believe,
Have I a choice
For I hear your voice
Then with my pen
I pull up my sleeves
Shall I not do what I can?
I will do it to please
Until your voice should cease
I could
Do your slightest desire
You are the wood
I am the fire
I have your eyes
Inside of my head
I must not lie
I have not led
Myself this far
It is just that my senses
You constantly jar
The love that you smell
Is also in my nostrils
Your touch
Is such
A feeling
Of healing
Your taste
Is as sweet tarts
Making haste to depart.

LETTERS TO LEIGH

And help myself to love

I would not
Be here
If I did not
Love you, dear
I would not care
Where you are
Yet I do
I love you,
Whatever else does come
Along
Only makes me more
Willing to wait on the love-store
To open
Its door,
I am hoping
Someone else will lose
His key
I would cover it with my shoes
Hurriedly
Then when down I bent
To pick it up
My hands would make a double-cup
For I should think that it is heaven sent
I would not
Nor could not
Put it into my pocket
I would place it within the locket
Give the door a shove then help myself to love.

LETTERS TO LEIGH

I shall be loving you

When you go home
I shall be loving you
When you are in his arms
I will be loving true
When you are awake
My love I shall take
Then upon the wind
I will send my thoughts for you that feel so good
Then in a similar way you should
Send
One
Back home
To me, friend
I shall keep what
You sent
As that
Heaven lent
For when
The day does wan
I will take your love
Sent from above
Inside of my home
Where I will be alone
I shall still be feeling good
As I think that maybe I should
Ask for you from God
Yet instead I just nod.

LETTERS TO LEIGH

To begin a love letter

I am still
Going to write you letters
Until
My heart does feel better
Yet I am going to write
In the light
That we have not ever been
Separated then
As we one day
Come together to stay
 we shall uncover
These letters of each others
We will be right on time
With our rhyme
It will change our sulk
Into laugh and talk
A smile you shall have
Slowly turning into a laugh
While upon my chin
I will bear a big grin
We shall laugh and shake
Until it is late
Then I will turn the lights down
While you put on your gown,
Since the children are fed
We shall jump into bed
To begin a love letter
In a way that is better.

LETTERS TO LEIGH

By my soul fed

My heart jumped
Today
Then a lump
Found the lonely way
Into my throat
 I hoped
The vision
That I was seeing
Had a mission
Of relieving
Then of healing
This bad feeling
That you were lost,
Tho I paid the cost,
Of coming here
Without fear
Of my own sake
Only to take
Your image,
At this stage,
Into my heart
Then start
It on its way
Up to my head
To there stay
By my soul fed
Today my heart leaped
As forever then in love it was steeped.

LETTERS TO LEIGH

For just a few moments more

I watched you from
The window
As I leaned upon
My elbow
You were walking
Around and talking
To folks resting,
Like eggs nesting,
Then you moved on
Looking for someone
Tho you could not find
Whom you had in mind
After a time
You made a line
Toward
The door
I had a look
Then I took
A walk
To see if I may talk
With someone
Alone,
I looked through the door,
I would have swore
That you were waiting
For me to walk in
Yet I watched you through the door
Then my heart watched just a few moments more.

LETTERS TO LEIGH

As long as we are together

I shocked you today
As your arm lay
Touching mine,
I noticed that you did not whine
You have shocked me so
Often I know
What it feels
Like to touch a real
Live wire,
Tho I never tire
Or fail to appreciate
While you like to negotiate
Terms of surrender
To bring an end to the sweet torture,
Yet such accidents
Are hard to prevent
For try as I may
Here your arms lay
Again
To be shocked when
Our skin misses
As our hair kisses
So forgive me, dear
If as your arm does lay near
We shock each other
It is due to the weather
For as long as we are together
We will just forgive one another.

LETTERS TO LEIGH

Myself alone

I was not going to ask for a kiss
It is just not that I am willing to miss
One, I only thought,
While in my mind I fought
Myself alone
To keep from giving you oneac
While we stand and wait
 Near the gate
Of what is good
With a thought of what we should
Be doing since
Our wooing went
Into despairs door
What is more
I am not sure
Anymore
Of how to woo
You or how to do
Any romance,
I cannot leave it to chance,
Yet my best bet
Would be to let
You know that
I do not know what
To say or do
Or even to make a move
Because I was gonna ask of you for more than a
kiss,
It is a chance that I am not willing to miss.

LETTERS TO LEIGH

Happy you should be

You do not have to be cruel
Tonight
You could let your heart rule
Perhaps it yet might
You do not have to act aloof
The look in your eyes is the proof
You do not have to sit so far away
You could pull up close and stay
Should you not have something to say?
A few words, anyway,
There are people around, so pray,
For maybe they will not go on their way
I do not know why you should not talk
I have never known you to sulk
Happy you should be;
You will be far away from me,
Since I am the cause of so much trouble
I would be out of here upon the double
Yet I know from the way that you are acting
Your love I am extracting
Even though we are apart in your mind
That thought will be proven only by time
If we sit apart
That would still only start
Our heart to pulsing
Then our love to coursing
There is not any need for us to be fools
Nor for us to be cruel
Let us just move our stools.

We may mend our sweet sorrow

You shall be leaving tomorrow
Then bequeathing to me sorrow
I shall have not a place to borrow
Happiness tomorrow
Yet happy
I do want you to be
I would rather like for you to be glad
Not to wish that you had
Stayed here
To see my tear
Fall
 That is not all
You surprise me so often
Each time that you come suddenly,
As my eyes you do soften,
Upon me
Even though I like it
I am surprised quite a bit
Because forever I am pleased by you,
That is so true
Yet that is not why
 I wish to say good-bye
The reason is this,
The season to kiss
Is past
Now at last
We may mend our sweet sorrow
The day following tomorrow.

LETTERS TO LEIGH

I am still not believing

I did not know when I met you
That you would forget that you know
Me, yet I think it now
Tho I cannot see how
 You should ever do
This to a love that is so true
It is almost as hard to stand by
 As it is not to cry
When now that you are leaving
I am still not believing
How you are treating
My friendly greeting,
Yet you just stand there
As if you do not know where
We have ever met
Or how did I get
The idea that you would
Or even that you should
Treat me, poor clod,
As other than as some poor piece of sod
Intended for you to place under-foot
Or to maybe my heart uproot
Then stamp upon
While you just put your foot down
On and politely excuse your-self
That due to your health
You just cannot stand
Any demand
Then command
Me to be an ex-friend.

LETTERS TO LEIGH

Before we part

I know not why I keep writing to you
You do not love me, it is true,
I do not love you, so,
That is a lie, I do
For I would be a fool
Not to do
Homage at your stool
My wish and my hope
Is for you to cope
With this feeling
That this love is sealing
Within our heart
Before we part
Tho my love is impaired
By your love it shall be repaired
Then in the end
Love will send
Loves medicine
To cure the cracks within
Our heart
For love will start
To grow again
 Then
We shall each
 The other teach
Courses at home,
 Keeping our love strong.

LETTERS TO LEIGH

You turned with that stare

What does hurt most
Is the friendship lost,
The thought of waking up and knowing
That your smile is somewhere showing
Those little moments
That to miss are torment
Like the glances that we gave one another outside
walking around
Over the half-frozen ground
Watching the birds return
From their winter sojourn
Then at a picnic table sitting down
Waiting for that familiar frown
That you would often lose
As we would talk and you used
The back of your head
When we speak of our love as dead
Yet then as you would turn around
 I would know that our love was safe and sound
Suddenly you would get up then I would follow
Back where we sat we had left our sorrow
Then you must have needed one drink more
For, indeed your throat does seem to be sore
Then a coat you wished that you had worn
So we headed on toward the dorm
Tho before
We were there
You turned with that stare
In one another's reflection we both had hidden
tears.

LETTERS TO LEIGH

Mine own that was not ever left behind

Were you lying
With your sighing
I cannot believe it
It just does not fit
You felt love and more
When I walked through the door
You gave to me a smoke
 then you made a joke
I was shy
Although you put me on a mental high
Then you gave me to know
Softly, that you had a great soul
Then as I did my part
My love did start
To trap me, as if your heart had cobwebs
Wherein I fell, into your hearts bed
Until like a black widow
I would have died to be your fellow
I found that you had a fine brain
More a-likened to a hurricane
For when something made you frown
It was as if you just blew it down
Yet sometimes you just went around
With a head full of steam on your way to give
sound
Tho your heart
Would start
To keep in mind
Mine own that was not ever left behind.

LETTERS TO LEIGH

I look into your eyes

Now that you have gone
Having left me all alone
I still see your face
Although it is only a trace
Just a flash now and then
With a smile or a grin
Giving me a greeting
On my coming or leaving
Then when I open a door
My spirits do soar
For while my hearts eye does blink
I seem to think
You are still here
Not there
Then with a spring to my step
While love is in the depth
Of my heart
I am in part
Ready to go on my way
Yet the rest of me would like me to stay
 To help me decide
I look into your eyes
Yet they always say
Be on your way
For now
This is how
I have gotten around
Since you have left town.

LETTERS TO LEIGH

I shall be in preparation

Just in time
I saw you leaving
Now I am grieving
Heart and mind
I waved come back
Do not leave yet
There is not any lack
Of eyes that are wet
Well, then I sat down
Into a chair
Alone with my frown
 I kind of messed with my hair
I thought it all over
Squared up both shoulders
All nice and tight
Then calmed my mind to settle down for the long
fight
Until slowly upon me it dawned
Somehow I was shown
That this was only a battle lost
Not so much in the wars final cost
 I gathered my somewhat questionable forces
Checked all of my unknown resources
Then chose to engage my foe that I had to beat
By waging war in retreat
For while he has to keep up,
Feed and shine my love cup
I shall be in preparation
By collecting loves ammunition.

LETTERS TO LEIGH

She has my heart

I want my baby back
I want her now
I care not for tact
I care not how
She has my heart
Torn into two parts
I do not mind sharing
Only for her I am caring
I want my woman
All safe and sound
Shall tender thoughts from this hand
Bring her around:
I want thee kind Leigh
With tender and care
May I on bended knee
Kiss thy hair
To me come back early
I am able to cherish thee
More than diamonds and pearl
I have asked for thee on bleeding knee
My heart has fallen unto thee
Lady McFall, to my heart thou art near
Than all
 Ransom love, say yea to mine ear
 Come back to me feyish fairy queen Haynes
My love for thee is just right
 What this heart speaks shall cause thee not pain
 Hasten with thy glow into my sight.

LETTERS TO LEIGH

Do anything for you that I could

I am sitting on the spot
Where we would often stop
 Here we often sat
This is where we often chat
I always sat on your right
Forever keeping you in sight
You always sat on my left
Taking your kisses by theft
Then we arose to walk around
With both your eyes upon the ground
Now we walked opposite
I on your left, you on my right
Yet I would just smile and walk on
Not once giving you a reason to frown
Your pocketbook was quite a load
For then you decided that we would hit the road
Toward the door
From there up to fourth floor
 to talk and smoke some more
Where I was never bored
Then as you would have a drink
 I would take time to think
About this new thing that I had found
To keep the mind sane and sound
I would put it into a can
Wherein it should benefit man
Yet just now I know that I would
Do anything for you that I could.

LETTERS TO LEIGH

I miss you now as then

These people do seem to be so wishy-washy
 Often they do seem to be so flip-floppy
Do not try to make them friends
Or with your heart you may make amends
I do not see how
I do put up with them now
Or how you did the days
That I was gone away
I miss you now as then
I do not know how you have been
Are you keeping fit
Whether or not if you are being hit
I hope that you are staying fed
Do you plan to wed
Are you still wearing pink
Maybe you are at the kitchen sink
Perhaps you are looking
For what you may have planned on cooking
Or if you have taken
A notion to do some baking
My heart just does not know
I have yet to be told
How you have been,
For I have just not seen
You for days
Now I pray
That your heart you shall lend
To me your friend.

LETTERS TO LEIGH

Everywhere that I go

I am just sitting outside
Watching the wind ride
Around and around
Then all about town
Here is an empty seat
I think that it would be neat
If you were sitting near
Then my love would rear
For I hold you dear
With me you are without peer
These people are talking about cooking,
As for me, I am only looking
At your ghost
That to me does play host
While it puts on a show
Everywhere that I go
Now they are speaking of wine
Yet it cannot be as fine
As the vintage that I drink
When to my knees I sink
As I pray to God
Upon humble sod
That one day I may take
You for my wife to make
 my whole life I will stake
For your sake
Then one flesh we shall be
 Within all eternity.

LETTERS TO LEIGH

How deep my love does go

I shall take this empty page
Then add words that will gauge
How deep my love does go
Forever how my heart should know
That you are she
Who does make me weak at the knees
With this pen
I shall send
Up smoke signals
That will lull
You into a daze
Then that loving gaze
Will look into mine
As I for always then shall know that I will walk the
line
With my hand I pledge
Also my heart does allege
That I love you
With a love that is true,
From these eyes that are seeing
Including all of my being
I promise you today
My heart upon a tray
For you to abuse
Or misuse
As long as you choose
This heart of a fools
It is yours for the taking
Please do not take it for breaking.

Just hold me

Just hold me
Do not scold me
Just hold me
Yes, boldly
You take all of my fear
When you hold me near
Left in its place
I have your face
For my comfort then my cheer
You are so, so dear
I love you most
When you are my host
For pleasant company
You shall always be
We may hold hands
Or walk in the sand
Then lay around
Upon the ground
Tho it may be best
If we take our rest
Inside of the house
As man and spouse
To there start the game
That ends the same
With loving laughter
After
All of the outside fun
Is done.

LETTERS TO LEIGH

Of the broken heart that we then had

I will be ready
 Calmly holding steady
Waiting on my friend,
Her heart she shall lend,
For she will be glowing
With the knowing
That has led
Toward our being wed
Yet we shall go slow
For she does know
Procrastination
Builds anticipation
 That happy feeling
Gives to broken hearts a healing
 She will of that be needing
Not her grief to be feeding
Then one day she will look back
Forever to be amazed at the knack
Of how we fell in love with ease
Just as pretty as you please
While the years go by
Then as time begins to fly
We will both be glad
Of the broken heart that we then had
Which our love mended
From our hearts that tended
To come together for life
Becoming loving man and wife.

LETTERS TO LEIGH

Like an ocean at low tide

I shall be waiting,
Anticipating,
Daydreaming
Scheming
Then yearning
To be learning
If you are ready
To go steady
If you will give that soft hand
To me as a friend,
If you shall spend you life
As my wife,
If ever there was a need
For such a good deed
The time is now
Yet take your time, anyhow
It is not my aim to rush
Only just to give a gentle push
You I shall wait to be delivered
By the aid of cupids quiver
I want you to gently slide
Into my arms opened wide
Please do not your deep feelings try to hide
Like an ocean at low tide
For as we watch each others eyes
The tide will gently start to rise
 When the tide is high again
Loves sweet emotion will begin.

LETTERS TO LEIGH

Love that will stay

I am outside today
Watching people as they play
A game with gloves
Tho I am waiting on love
They have bats
Yet I have that
Which is above all
A loving ball
 I shall watch
Then I will catch
Each one thrown
 For let it be known
That I shall take home
Every one
Which does come my way
After that I shall lay down my glove
Only when it is full of love,
Love that will stay,
Will I not catch all of that love
With my glove
I shall catch it all
I will not fall
Shall I not take it home
Where I am alone
Tho if I need love
I will look to my glove
 Then anon,
I shall just put it on.

LETTERS TO LEIGH

I know that you love me true

I do not know how I made it
All of those years
How could I just sit
Then waste my tears
A whilst I was growing up
 On my heart to sup
When all of the while
You were only a few mile
Away
Where you were likely to stay
Unknown to me
Until we
Both came down
With the same frown
Yet we let
That go and met
Each others grin
Then we became each others friend
I love you
I know that you love me true
What more could I ask
Than for that special task
Instead of years that are wasted
I will treat the past as days that I have tasted
Of life without Leigh
Then we shall have found that they weigh
A very small amount
Compared to our new love fount.

LETTERS TO LEIGH

Is your heart to haunt?

I have the angel's hand
That holds the magic wand
 Which changes anything
Or happiness may bring
Anytime that I choose
To use
My beautiful mind
To do something kind
What I really want
Is your heart to haunt
From this ink that has fell
Into your mind to dwell
 As these words gently flow
I want to know your soul
Is it white
I shall not dye it
Yet I will blend
In as a friend
Then whatever shade
That will be made
Will be great
If I am not too late
I will be on time
To add mine
To yours
 For then ours
Will be a new
And beautiful hue.

LETTERS TO LEIGH

Just hold me close and near

I just want you
To be as much in love with me
As I am such in love
With ye
I do not know
Why, I just do
Yet let me seek to say,
Maybe I should attempt this way,
Let me put it in a song
Just do not tell me that I am wrong
My love for you is as strong
As my love for you is long
Loving is caring
 Caring is sharing
Sharing is loving
Without pushing and shoving
If I want some love I will ask
As you want some, such an easy task
I shall love you long and dear
Just hold me close and near
All the rest
We will go past
On our quest
To make love last
 As we reach the end
We shall both stand
Then receive a hand
Up into the Promised Land.

LETTERS TO LEIGH

To make you my own

My heart is in flames
My soul is the timber
The heat is reaching my brain
As I try to remember
Just what am I doing
Loving and wooing
Another mans woman
 Just how do I plan
To make you my own
When I am not known
To lie, cheat, or steal
Yet now I appeal
For I am willing
To attempt love stealing
For what should be stolen
Would be who I was once holding
 To have you back
I would open my sack
Of young woman lures
Until I found all of the cures
That you badly need
For which my heart does bleed
Please do not ask how I could do this
It is easy, especially for bliss
What joy I brought to you then
Will grow and multiply when
You have caught yourself on my hook
When I have regained what he took.

LETTERS TO LEIGH

All of my thoughts are safe with you

I do not want you saying
That I was not there
When you know that I am praying
Even from here
I pray for happiness in your life
Tho I hope that one day you shall be my wife
If that sounds confusing
Just consider the bruising
That I myself take
As my prayers and hopes do make
For me a divided soul
Yet I know that I may be whole
For you will have a happy life
Living as my wife
My soul does not have to be torn in two
For I know that all of my thoughts are safe with
you
I do not have to slip and slide
Because one day you shall be my bride
 Then when you are such
I shall finally touch
All of those secret places
Then let down your silk laces
My hands will be lost in your hair
As my eyes shall be lost in your stare
My arms themselves will hold your back
Until nothing there is to lack
Except across your lips
 Soon to them I will have placed my fingertips.

LETTERS TO LEIGH

There are thoughts hidden

All of my dedications
 with my heartfelt illustrations
Do not dare
Ask that I share
My feelings so fine and fair,
I just cannot commit
My pen to submit
Any words that I shove
Onto this paper
As the words of love
That in my heart capers,
You I do love
 within my hearts cove
There are thoughts hidden
That I cannot keep the lid on
One glance at you and my heart stands still
My blood beats faster as my eyes drink their fill
From you one touch
Does affect my love as such
That I would do any task
Anything, anything that you should ask
Just touch my lips with yours
That I may reach loves shores
 should our bodies gently swell
We will be in a sweet, silent hell
All these tender thoughts I forever save
For your hand within mine I shall always crave.

LETTERS TO LEIGH

Yet when we meet then

I miss you baby
I miss your face
I miss you lady
In this place
I need you Leigh
You need me
When I leave here
We will meet somewhere
We have had near misses
With our kisses
Yet when we meet then
We shall stay chin to chin
Will we not have a drink
Then have time to think
Of where we will go
What we shall do
I will be ready
To hold you steady
As I play rock-a-bye-baby
With you, my lady
I shall lay my head within your lap
While my hands give you gentle slaps
We shall finally pull back the cover
 I will rub your back over and over
When it is time we shall turn out the light
Soon to gently make love the rest of the night
Early morning finally brings rest
I will miss you baby, our love is of the best.

LETTERS TO LEIGH

I will take your hand in mine again

You were not wearing
That wedding band
Are you still caring
To share my hand
You are she
Who makes me feel like a man
I am he
That made your blood ran
If we ever
Get together
I shall be your pillow
 then your fellow
You will be my girl
For you I shall swirl
Around the room
Until you swoon
I will lay you down upon the divan
Then I shall take you up to heaven
Among the clouds we will go prancing
Our hearts themselves shall feel like dancing
We will let each other come down slowly
Shall we not be feeling kind of holy
When our feet touch the ground
You shall be ready for another round
I will take your hand in mine again
 that is the sign to begin
As we rise hand in hand
You shall have on my wedding band.

LETTERS TO LEIGH

Anytime day or night

You are not talking
To me now
You are not balking
Nor have forgotten how
It is just that
We cannot chat
For I shall be a little
Longer in the hospital
Yet I will soon not be here
Then I shall welcome all of your cheer
Your call will be a welcome delight
Anytime day or night
When your voice I do here
I shall close my eyes then think that you are near
After I have closed my eyes for awhile
I will break into a great big smile
While we are talking I shall get on my knees
Then give thanks to God for answering me
I shall then lay down on the floor
How do I know, I have done so before
The time will come to say good-bye
Then I shall pick the line back up and say hi
All I will hear is the dial tone
 I shall hang up and talk to no one
Then my happiness I will keep inside
Until in someone I shall have to confide
I guess there is no tone nearer
Than for me just to tell my mirror.

LETTERS TO LEIGH

Love that waits upon a rainy day

You are a rainy day woman
Sometimes you are torn
Between sunshine and rainy days
Yet you will find your way through the maze
A fine example you would make
For all the other women who take
The long way to have
Then hold their special love
Because you will eventually find the way
I am saving my love for that rainy day
All of the same I do hope and pray
That you soon find the way that does pay,
You I shall wait here to greet
While silently wish that you could cheat
Maybe I know that you must pass this test
Before your soul may find sweet rest
You must explore every route
Until you find that you are safely out
I did not want you in this mess
Tho it may be for the sake of goodness I must
confess
When it is all said and done
You may tell him that you have won
Whether or not I win or lose
That is still for you to choose
Yet do not let your eyes grow wet
Because still hope is not over yet
For love is here, love that stays
Love that waits upon a rainy day.

LETTERS TO LEIGH

If only I may be a friend

In my heart
I know that you are mine
If you would only start
To just read between the lines
I have followed you from floor to floor
Holding open all of the doors
Toward the chapel you I have led
Although we were never wed
I have loved you since first sight
When we met that dark night
My good love kept on growing
As your qualities you kept on showing
Then one day you asked for a ring
What happened soon after, only three did I bring
You then tried them on
As you said that you would provide the wedding
gown
Later we talked about kids
I said that I would be father to his
Then one thing led to another
We decided that I would be your brother
I knew that our relationship I could mend
If only I may be a friend
I went away for a little while
Yet I came back to find your smile
I do not know how it should be worded
Although it seemed to me that me you avoided
That is alright, I do not read signs
For in my heart I know that you are mine.

LETTERS TO LEIGH

The wind and the rain

It just happened
I cannot explain
Who should separate
The wind and the rain
Who would divide
Sorrow and pain
Does anyone know what it may feel like
For the pools of love to flood the hearts dike
 as love, as love does in that way come rushing
down
Upon the love starved ground
Causing love to flower
Then urgent love to tower
Above lesser emotions
While the faint-hearted notions
That cannot find their way
tend to just stay
Sitting on the floor
Or hiding behind the door
That leads to life
Away from silly strife
Tho do not ask me, I am only a poet
When it comes to love, I do not know it
I have looked high and I have looked low
Yet I guess I have been just too slow
One day I shall find it and I will know when
Because I shall never have to look for it again
For it is like the wind and like the rain
Full of sorrow, full of pain.

LETTERS TO LEIGH

Yet the silence does fill my ears

You had me eating
Out of your hand
You had me sweating
 the teardrops ran
You had control over all of my thoughts
Control over my own I had naught
That face stayed with me all day long
At night I dreamed to the sound of your song
I would awaken with blood on fire
Of dreams of you I could never tire
Then I would get back in bed between the sheets
 to there face alone the heat
Morning comes, I awaken at dawn
To find new thoughts your dream has sown
I take the sheets from around my thighs
Blink twice and open my eyes
Then I thought that I heard you call my name
Once again my heart is in flames
All alone I call your name, Leigh, please be mine,
I shall love you until the end of time
Yet the silence does fill my ears
 as my hands are filled with tears
Then I prepare to face the day
Another day without the face of Leigh
Evening comes and I am all prepared
To meet you in my dreams if we dare
I lay down in bed then for you I await
Until love opens heavens gate.

LETTERS TO LEIGH

Only time may tell

I can sense
That something has changed
Maybe chance
Has rearranged
Something in my life
Causing so much strife
Maybe the time has come
For me to think of coming home
To a wife and child
Both so sweet and mild
Only time may tell
If to Leigh I will kneel
Tho I plan for right now
To be wondering how
I could deserve this
Newly found bliss
When I have always been
Such a loner, lonely man
Yet I will not tell where I have been
Nor ask her to say what she has seen
Past is past, best forgotten
Just think of our newly begotten
Then of the day that he will start kindergarten
I do not want to recall anything rotten
As we go through life
We shall have each other
Then we will give him strife
With a sister and brother.

LETTERS TO LEIGH

An emotional healing

God is teaching
Man is preaching
About love
How it is above
Ordinary feelings
An emotional healing
You do not know what you are missing
If, like some, you frown on kissing
Take it from me, find you a lady
Then you and her may be kissing steady
If her heart you hope to win
Just realize that to kiss is not a sin
My lady has lips so fine
I think that I am kissing sugar wine
Just remember not to slip
Just keep kissing on her lip
She shall take that as a sign
That you are willing to walk the line
After awhile, after she rest
She shall want you to hold her breast
As her breast you hold so near
She will keep thinking dear, oh dear
Then she shall cause your hand to slip
A little lower to her hip
To you it has never felt so fine
 just wait for her next sign
Now you finally have your lady
Take both hands and love her madly.

LETTERS TO LEIGH

As I love you tenderly and dear

I wish that I could let you know
In just a few words or so
How I really love you true
  of all the things for you that I would do
I could never let you down
I would always be your clown
Your joy I would not ever drown
For tender love I hope to own
All your kisses I would take
Then love them all for your sake
My love for you I could never fake
Yet would add mine for our new life to make
I could not stand to let you cry
I would hold you close then ask you why
after all of your tears were dry
I would never tell you another lie
Should I not help you to clean the house
Like a loving spouse
Then after all of the kids were fed
We would talk of the day that we were wed
Out of the kitchen you go while me you led
Into the room that does hold our bed
I lay myself down upon the cover
You then come back then say move over
As I love you tenderly and dear
In the early morning I hold you near
As the sun must rise from the east
We heighten again to our love feast.

LETTERS TO LEIGH

Love is only one step away

Do not ask what I think you should do
There is a chance that I would make your heart
feel blue
Do not ask me to make a decision
That would slice through my heart like an incision
Ask me not if you should stay with him
For to me loves chances are pretty slim
yet I do think that you have never really given me
a chance
To choose me would only make sense
You need someone to appreciate
Those very fine and unique traits
Not someone that would bring you down
To ruin your name all over town
How many chances does he get
While I wait for you and yet
You do not give to me the time of day
Something should tell me that he does like it that
way
He has spat on you then knocked you around
while with me I have never seen you frown
Our love is living on borrowed time
Waiting on the clock-down-to-wind
Before the sand within my glass does touch the
bottom
I want to taste your love then taste it often
The time is now short
You do not always have to be a good sport
Just take the children and run,
Come right into my waiting arms
Please leave now, do not delay

LETTERS TO LEIGH

Love is only one step away.

LETTERS TO LEIGH

True love is not ever wrong

I love you Leigh
Do you understand
What love may be
Between a woman and a man
 thy love is crazy
My love is lazy
Willing to wait
On heavens gate
To open the way
Where then my heart will stay
Never to depart
From where love does start
I love you Leigh
Do not make me bleed
Too, too much
Awaiting on thy touch
Just touch me with soft love
 give to my heart a gentle shove
Just tell me where to stay
 I shall never go away
I love you Leigh
Thou were meant for me
  please always be mine
Until the end of time
Do not make me wait too long
I am a fraught with sad songs
With me here is where you belong
True love is not ever wrong.

LETTERS TO LEIGH

When I have part of you to feel

We will be surprised
When next we see us
A tear will be prised
If we meet at the bus
A smile is what we shall see
As we sit by a tree
If we could only touch now
We would see how
That we
Are meant to be
I will feel good when
Gently I may touch you again
Although I felt better
To find your letter
I shall feel better still
When I have part of you to feel
It does not matter, just any part,
That is just where I will start
To stroke
Until you are broke
Yet are ready then
To be put together again
For I shall be ready
To start all over
While holding you steady
I may start on your shoulder
Until you are ready
For me to grow bolder.

LETTERS TO LEIGH

Then unto me you may give your deepest emotion

I have almost ran out of words
Yet that does not mean that I do not care
I say that I have almost ran out of verbs
Although that does not mean that my heart does
not tear
When I think of the love that I have lost
Words more or less do not add much to the cost
Of losing a love so true
Which is to say that I am losing you
Tho I have not yet began to fight
Because my true love was once in sight
I shall not let love turn out its light
Just because it is loves darkest night
I will fight on while the battle rages
Laying my love down on these pages
They shall be there for you to read
When your heart is ready for me to lead
I will retreat only as far as I must
To steal your heart from among the dust
I will have you to love and to hold
I shall just have to let my heart grow bold
Kissing both hands, I shall kneel at your feet
There I will give to you kisses that are so sweet
To you I shall give all of my devotion
Then unto me you may give your deepest emotion
I will take you home to be my wife
You shall come to see that I have saved your life
Please come to believe that you may have been
wrong
Because by my side is where you belong.

LETTERS TO LEIGH

A loving fool

I miss you
never may I replace
You baby
 the trace
Of my tear
Is falling I fear
Out of my eye
To be near my smile
I tell you not a lie
Knowing not am I guile
Am I faking
This teardrop that you are making
Because I do miss you so
How many tears will fall
I just do not know
 yet fall they shall
Until they accumulate
A small pool
To accentuate
A loving fool
I am heavy hearted
As I am so easily startled
I cannot keep going
With wet eyes showing
It is you that I want to date
I do not care if it is now late
Only you may dry my eyes
Then please soothe my ears with your soft sighs.

LETTERS TO LEIGH

I love you Leigh

Dear Leigh,
How are you
Do you have anything to say
Are you feeling blue
I miss you Earle
I ever want you for my girl
Shall I not waste away while
I am waiting on your special smile
I do not want you me to fear
Tho you are beautiful in tears
could not you let me dry your eyes
You should give to me your soft sighs
I just want to make you laugh,
Laugh and laugh until you cough
Until your sides wiggle
then until you giggle
I want to let the good times roll
Then roll through you into your soul
Until these good things take their toll
To give you back what someone stole
I love you Leigh, do not forget
never allow your heart to let
Any doubt of me to sneak in
To do so would surely be a sin
I do not judge anyone
Just please do not leave me all alone
I love you Leigh.
Please do not leave me.

LETTERS TO LEIGH

Where cupids arrow aimed

I was there
Now I am here
Only my tear
I need to fear
What I am hearing
Is your voice searing
Into my ears
As my soul does tear
I pick up the halves
To apply love salve
Unto my broken soul which may then become one
tho alone
Yet it begins to feel better
As I read that last letter
Now my eyes are even wetter
While my heart is in fetters
I take up the chain
That has me in pain
I read it again
Then my heart does become tame
Although it is still maimed
Where cupids arrow aimed,
I pull that out
Now there is a fount
Of love gushing from
Where the arrow did come
I know that you are not a bum
Yet may I please offer you some.

LETTERS TO LEIGH

Tis love at first sight

Now this is what I do have to offer
For you should know that I am a pauper
I offer to you love on a silver platter
All of this love yet never grow fatter
Except that your soul may tend to grow big
As you feast on loves juicy figs
That is just an illustration
Now feel your hearts palpitations
As the more that I write
The greater the height
Will fly your love kite
For tis love at first sight
Not again will you need other guys
You will never begin to hear more lies
Because now that you have nix
You will always be up late
For I think of tricks
Then play them straight
Now I do not intend to boast
Yet I fully intend to play host
With your love then soon I shall coast
On to the part that you love most
Please allow me to put it in a plain word,
You are the sheath, I am the sword
I will regain you whatever the cost
I shall regain your love that is lost.

LETTERS TO LEIGH

You know me Leigh

Baby I have heard the spirits
Be still, may it be that you feel it
They are saying there is peace here
So dry your eye and calm your fear
They say here is where you belong
To talk your talk and sing your song
The bees are out
The birds are singing
There is a water fount
 the bells are ringing
For us to marry
So why tarry
where you are
With heart scarred
That tender soul mangled
Often soft emotions tangled
Come and follow me
together we
May make a brand new start
For love will restore your heart
You know me Leigh
Can you not see
That our love is grand
So let us join hands
Then let us be rash
Let us make a dash
Toward happiness
Which is the spice of life, more or less.

LETTERS TO LEIGH

Yet when I am all alone

I just have to be near you Leigh
For there is still a chance that we
May friends and lovers be
Let me help your eyes to see
That I am the only one
Who must feel that forever with your past you may
be done
me you cannot do wrong
join hands with me and come along
My hands are big while yours are strong
Joined together they belong
Yet when I am alone
My hands do seem to lose their tone
I am kind of sick while sort of weak
 my hands do seem to grow kind of meek
I think of you, that then does help some
For my hands then do remember all of the fun
That they had once then they are stunned
for now your memory again does burn
As my hands take a turn
Trying to write down
What your memory has sown
I love you Leigh
Please, believe me
My hand will never harm
nor feel a cause to ever alarm
except to ransom your smile from a frown
To you whom our love has shown
That together we belong
Any other would be wrong.

LETTERS TO LEIGH

From me into your heart to stay

I miss you
Like the deserts miss the rain
I miss you
Like sorrow misses pain
I miss you Leigh
I know that you miss me
Just call me on the phone
When you are all alone
No one will ever know
There is not any evidence to show
A waiting at the other end
my pure love I do you send
We do not have to talk for long
I would like to hear you sing your song
Just talking cannot be wrong
maybe I shall sing along
How many times must I say
That you make my blues to go away
I love you Leigh, that is true
Please, just do not be too cruel
Pick up the phone then call me today
Just please, oh please do not delay
We shall see if love finds the way
From me into your heart to stay
There it is bound to show
Where it is bound to grow
My heart does miss you Leigh
Just call me, please.

LETTERS TO LEIGH

Around my heart

Now that I am home
I know where love does come from
For I have seen
That love surely must come from where I have
been
I would like to do it all again
Maybe then I would win
I had won you then I lost you fair
Now I am only holding thin air
Where once you did belong
Now there is just what is left of your song
That you used to me sing
As you turned and turned your ring
Leigh, I love you
You may bet that it is true
What more could a fool
Ever possibly do
Than to write you these letters
As I hope to feel better
By using this pen
Hoping to lend
To this paper
A love that ever does caper
Around my heart
With a fire trying to start
Inside of my soul
Which is not quite whole
Because like my heart
You took a part.

LETTERS TO LEIGH

Of from where love pours

I carry thoughts around
Inside of my head
I listen to sounds
Then to what is said
Sometimes they help me to say
What is on my heart anyway
The sum of all does help my brain to shove
Forth these thoughts of love
I may have happened to tell you once
I should have told you before
All of these poems
Because you are who I so adore
Are yours, my Leigh
 I believe
That we will never be apart
When love starts
To pull open the door
Of from where love does pour
All of my bad emotions down I do lay
Now I await on what you shall say
When you have the feeling that only love does pay
Only love willing to stay
Away from you, far away
Until your love does to forever say okay
Then while your eyes look into mine
Looking for loves true signs
I will then stand there tall and I shall
Of your love be waiting to take it all.

LETTERS TO LEIGH

The sounds of our heart are forever sealed

We are young
We are not old
We are strong
Now let us be bold
To touch
A love of such
Pure feeling
That our hearts
Will start
To feel the healing
Of that I need some
I know you do too
Let us take it from me and you
I love you Leigh
Just touch me please
I shall take my turn
Your heart I would not ever burn
Yet should I not give an alarm
That would save you from harm
To save you from life's storms
Then would I encircle you until the coming morn
For then I should wake up to have you to hold
 have we not sought then found and bought love
and sold
Then knowing forever that we have a goodly deal
The sounds of our heart are forever sealed
Have my love for an eternal age
We have swapped love for love at a most sweet
manner of wage.

LETTERS TO LEIGH

Must be that I shall not ever erase

Would I lie
To you baby
Would I lie
To you Leigh
You know me
Better than I know you
You should know if my
Lies are true
I have told you before
That I do not intend to make your heart sore
Yet have you even ever let,
On my account, your eyes to grow wet
I love you with a capital I
Please, you must tell
If these feelings that you feel
Do not or do tend to heal
Your broken heart
If it should start
To feel better
With each lying letter
The conclusion of the case
Must be that I shall not ever erase
My loving lies
From your ears to your eyes
I love you Leigh
Yet do I lie
Allow love to stay
Perhaps a little while.

LETTERS TO LEIGH

May be that one day I shall be whole

Oftentimes I have waken up
Late within the night
then I silently sup
From loves tender bite
I seem to taste love bit by bit
slowly, finally, up I then sit
Until my feet are softly wooing the floor
I press down on them for loves sweet feelings I
cannot ignore
This sweetest of love that is never ending
Has this poor heart ever bending
Love to you I love to keep on lending
Your timely payments there-of to me keep on
mending
A broken heart and soul
Have I not pleaded for your total that I might be
whole
In not any form should I slumber and sleep
I needs must to arise early for words of love come
not cheap
All who are needy must pay the timely price
Yea, stout heart beats and breaks the silence
When all goodly men find a chest of treasure, at
such he does prise
The possessor of that chest sets loves price then
the wise man buys
For to have the jewels offered by love, should we
not enter
With foolish key, toward the centre
Of a lady lost heart

LETTERS TO LEIGH

Risky shame indeed if we know not from where
love does start
Nay this is not a riddle yet only a pauper in loves
rhyme
now, as ever, has brought me back to bedtime
To lay down alone and lonely once more
Until a dream of love awakens me from my floor.

LETTERS TO LEIGH

To you, little dove

God is protecting our love
From up on high above
Waiting to give a gentle shove
To you, little dove
 I am waiting on God to lead the way
for I am waiting to hear you say
That you love me so
Like you used to do
I am waiting on the look upon your face
That shall tell me that I have won loves sweet race
I am waiting on the touch of your hand
As together a fragile walk we took in the sand
I am waiting on your voice in my ear
As I would again often hold you near
I am waiting on the taste of your mouth
As it is a sweet love fount
I am waiting to again touch your soul
Maybe then mine will become whole
I am waiting for the look in your eye
I had often looked yet did not ever find a lie
I am waiting for the touch of your breath
To soften the marks of love that your lips have left
I am waiting on you, to have then to hold
for my heart shall not ever grow cold
I am waiting to put my hands within your hair
As I slowly kiss you and hold you there
I am waiting on God above
Maybe he will let us love.

LETTERS TO LEIGH

Drinking in loves wine

I miss you Leigh
There is no doubt
That I do miss my sweet
Love fount
if I should ever come near to drink
I would take time to think
Then come to appreciate
Being so near to heavens gate
as your sweet water I start to taste
I would allow my heart to make haste
to drink all the love that it could
A knowing that it should
Not take a lonely time
Drinking in loves wine
At a time like this
My heart should only know bliss
Not to come near and miss
With a fizzle and a hiss
I do want to drink all that I can
For you are a love filled woman
before your love does wan
I do want to show that I am your man
I am coming near to drink you up
I am coming near to fill my cup
I am coming near to taste your spray
I am coming so near to your love to stay
I am ready for my love to flip-flop
I shall not ever be ready for your love to stop.

LETTERS TO LEIGH

For who may escape the power of love

I will stay in contact with Leigh
With what I like to call poetry
Writing to her, let me lead you unto paradise
 for once there I may see the blush of her eyes
To my ears would be her sighs
There her voice should pronounce not a lie
If I propose to make her mine
suppose that during this time
she would be ecstatic
Likely not, she may raise havoc
That is to be avoided at all cost
perhaps this would only be a battle lost
The next one fought,
Someday, is the one that I have longed for and
sought
There we will each
The other teach
A more tender flavour
Of loves wars to savour
For who may escape the power of love
Does not love give all a gentle shove
Into the way that is right
Looking not into all of the ways that are wrong
Yet seeing only where love alone is strong
If that is where you would like to fit
Make one more attempt,
To Levant
Your heart into loves gates to sit.

LETTERS TO LEIGH

Go ahead, give it some thought

Like a shadow, you follow me all of the time
You are before me with my rhymes
Without you I would be lost
Have I not already paid the cost
Please come along then hang around
We shall take a walk around loves grounds
Am I asking of you something that I should not
Baby, you should know if that happened then I
would be a wrought
All that the eye can see
I am willing to bestow toward loves fee
Go ahead, give it some thought
you will see what I have sought
For you are the one that I choose
All else, all else I am willing to lose
Except for me and you kissing
With hair tangled while our breath is hissing
What if forever-more
Love shuns away from your door
Who else should you open too
Would you let your heart grow blue
Now I am standing front and centre
Leave fickle heart bare then I shall enter
Through the doors of thy heart slightly left ajar
For that does aid and comfort myself from afar
As I would then the slightest of efforts have to use
In finding my lady love ever true
Once there we shall fall amidst the lucky clover
Better friend s yet and soon to be lovers.

LETTERS TO LEIGH

Amixing lonely ink with tears

A letter I held today
Thought I that it was from you, Leigh
Out came I and smiled
Felt I kind of like a child
Read I then the name
 it from someone else came
 me that still made happy
For did I in you believe
Wended I then on home
Opening the letter all alone
Followed me you there
Still with a perm in your hair
Then laid I the letter down
It was with my wits, gone
Of yourself thought I for awhile
Missed I especially your smile
Funny of face and all dimples
Just a grin, ah, simple
Moving thoughts toward your town
Afraid I would only make you frown
Guess I should stay just here
Amixing lonely ink with tears
Cadence of heart with memories sequence
Wish I that you were here
Would take you I then tear
Melodious love from your throat
As do I this envelope.

LETTERS TO LEIGH

You are still knocking on my loves doors

As I am writing on this ledger
I shall take time to pledge to her
That I love her true
For I am still her fool
Leigh, you must be thinking of me
My eyes are not playing make-believe
For everywhere that I go
Your face is sure to show
Whatever it is that you fear, your spirit
Does not fear it
It always finds a kind reception
Such a loved and sought for hallucination
Your face is always with me, Leigh
Always smiling, can you not see
You are with me even now
I feel you, true, yet I do not see how
It is you that does help me to write down
These words of love that your image has sown
You seem to want me to make a move
A move based on faith and trust in your love
To come to your town
to find your smile or frown
Yet if I come
Or if I stay at home
One thing is for certain, one thing is for sure
You are still knocking on my loves doors
I am going to find you, so goes the song
For I shall have that gentle spirit to help me along.

LETTERS TO LEIGH

What do I do now?

It is late at night and everyone is in bed
I am still thinking of what was said
The last time that we spoke
Love awoke
When you said that you would call
To save my heart from such a fall
I believed you and I still do
if you do not then I cannot sue
You for any love lost
Yet I will pay all of the cost
In more ways than one
As long as my heart is not alone
maybe you should know
That I may on your doorsteps one day show
To find out whether or not love is true
Or for love to make my heart turn blue
Tho you may make it red again
With just an easy laugh and a friendly grin
We could at least be one another's friend
With each others heart to lend
It should not have to end this way
We have ever not had enough to say
To be your dog you do not want me
As a friend you just cannot see
What do I do now
How do I find out how
Long I must wait
Until time opens heavens gate.

LETTERS TO LEIGH

Love is knocking at the door

People are going to jail
there are people going to hell
people are going upstairs
then there is me going not anywhere
In our love affair
I should have taken the stairs
Instead of waiting on the ride
They were there, just off to the side
This lack of exercise
Only gave rise
To time lost
With the later cost
Of losing you, Earle
My kingdom and my pearl
We ever had not time
To drink deeply of loves wine
Yet what I did taste
Made me to slowly make haste
To love you with all
My love and I shall
Be faithful to what I said
By the hair of my head
If it was only two weeks
It is love that now speaks
Speaks it what it spoke before;
Love is knocking at the door
Open up and let it in
Open up then let love win.

LETTERS TO LEIGH

Then her smile

You may only love so much
Without your lovers touch
When her hand is gone
You are left all alone
Her touch is all that you need
To plant loves seed
Her touch is all that you want
To open loves vault
Her touch is what you miss
The touch of her kiss
The touch of her can rend
The touch of her can mend
The touch of her can bend
The touch of her can send
You far away
Or near to stay
Just a simple gesture,
A touch of such texture
Does make me go wild
Or may gently keep me meek and mild
All of this love
Without her gloves
Just the tips of her fingers
Bid me to linger
A little while
then her smile
Commands me to stay
While her lips play.

LETTERS TO LEIGH

Loves seeds have been sown

I do not know what I am trying to say
I would give you my heart yet it is yours anyway
My heart, it is yours, yours to stay
For you my heart down I lay
Even with all of the lonely wounds
Even with all of them bound
It keeps on making the sound
Of a heart where love is found
What it is saying is true
For it says that I am in love with you
Always loving, never blue
Ever loving right on cue
All that is good and fine
Yet now I find that my heart repines
Because it failed to see the hidden signs
Down low is where it is lying
now is the time to raise it up
Toward your love it will sup
For your love will fill my hearts empty cup
Until its hup is back in fit stup
My heart is waiting all alone
Waiting for you to take it home
Your love is setting the tone
 I hurry before it is all gone
As you sat there in your gown
Toward you my love has flown
While now it has since shown
loves seeds have been sown.

LETTERS TO LEIGH

We hold our love in our hands

What would you say
If I took my love away
Or would it pay
Just to let it stay
Your soul I hope to touch
For that soul is such
An important thing
For it my own soul sings
A soft, soft song
Will not yours come along
We cannot be wrong
As our heart does beat that inner gong
While the rippling echoes
Light our fuse
that tells us soon
we shall be under the moon
Watching the stars
Compete from afar
all of their blinking
With our hidden winking
Has led me to thinking
That into love we are sinking
be that as it may
There is naught of time to delay
We hold our love in our hands
The clock is running out of sand
Let us open up your heart
Where love is sure to start.

LETTERS TO LEIGH

I love you Leigh, I am for real

What would you do
If my heart was torn in two
If I gave you the halves
Would you apply your love salve
I feel that is the case
When I look into your face
This feeling that I am feeling
Is my heart healing
For I have a feeling very far down
That one day in your love I shall be drowned
Then I will be found
Following your voice then your sound
I love you and by you will linger
You will not have to lift a finger
Just show me what you want
Then just stand aside, watch, and taunt
I shall do what you want me to
Anything that you want me to do
I love you Leigh, I am for real
My heart is bearing true loves seal
My love is such that I could kill
Anyone who would your love steal
My heart is ready for you to feel
Just take it in your hand then peel
Yet just take a little time
Because this heart that you hold is fine
Just taste this love for once
Before you get ready to pounce.

LETTERS TO LEIGH

I want you to know that I am waiting

With you I am on a natural high
I still hear your sigh
Then I know that it is not a lie
Even when it was time to say good-bye
I knew that we would be together again
The problem is that I do not know when
You may call me anytime
Tho I cannot call then change your mind
You may write to me any day
Yet you command my hand to stay
A word from you would bring a ray
Through the clouds your silence has delayed
If I ever hold you in my hands
I will know better than to make demands
I shall be happy just to be near
as you the direction of our life may steer
From me you will have nothing to fear
 I shall give you a smile in place of your tear
 I will try to guide you in this life
Away from anger and silly strife
For we need not be in a war
With feelings tangled then emotions tore
Shall we not be together to let love soar
Yes, we shall feel love in our hearts to the core
I want you to know that I am waiting
With hope in my eye and hearts blood sweating
I am doing nothing only anticipating
Our loves reconciliation.

All in due time

With ink on my hands
I humbly stand
With this wand
Inside of my palm
As I declare
That my love is fair
For he is holding you
Yet I am still true
For one day he will find out
That you are only my love fount
All in due time
When all of the wine
That he now may taste
Forever departs him in haste
To let me sup
From loves sweet cup
I have had to of love personally sacrifice
when he is without you of that he may have a slice
 I do know that sweet love I sorely have been missing
Perhaps you and I may soon be kissing
Even tho you are with him
I also know that his chances are pretty slim
Because in your dreams
I am in the scenes
While in the daytime
I am yet on your mind
Now I am waiting on the sign
Of forever that you will be mine.

LETTERS TO LEIGH

I shall find you one day

I still have not said all of what I want to say
We become close then we go away
One of us has to stay
For the other who has been delayed
Although your name is Earle
To me you shall always be of pearl
You are the one that I lost
At very great cost
the one that I have missed
That I have hugged then kissed
You are to be found somewhere,
Somewhere out there
I shall find you one day
I will never go away
I will be there to stay
Until I hear you say
Take my heart upon a tray
Take it now, do not delay
 I will take my own
Then beside yours lay it down
you could claim or disown
As long as love is sown
It shall fall on fertile hearts
into all of their fertile parts
as it moves within our veins
We will walk the lanes
Known as none other
Than as people who love one another.

LETTERS TO LEIGH

Never will we be afraid

If I were worthy of them
I would ask what your thoughts were
if they were of him
I could take my soul and tear
It apart
then take out my heart
pierce it with loves dart
To offer it up as a sweet tart
if you should touch it with your tongue
You would soak up love just like a sponge
Until you were dripping wet
Before you were nearly, nearly set
To be squeezed out
Making a love fount
For us to shower
Around loves tower
for us to climb down
Into the love that is sown
Then we shall shed tears
Because we have ended our fears
Never will we be afraid
Of what somebody has said
No more shall we have to peek
Or with love have to sneak
For when we are kissing
We will find that we are not missing
From getting caught
Yet that is loves fault.

LETTERS TO LEIGH

Into loves sweet hell

When we make love
Part of you will be in my veins
With loves gentle shove
You shall soon be feeling the same
Who would be better to share your blood
Than someone who always should
Agree with you in every way
To let you know loves here to stay
You should know yourself
That I just came off of the shelf
together we shall go well
at your feet I will kneel
Sweet words to you I shall tell
Until you hear loves bells
Into love I have fell
Into loves sweet hell
here is where I will pay
Here is where I shall lay
Here I will come to say
That to love I shall never say nay
Yet I will be there to lay you down
I shall be there to ease your frown
I will be there to hear your sound
I shall be there for your love to be drowned
In loves emotion
Adding to that our love lotion
For love makes you sore
Where twas not before.

LETTERS TO LEIGH

Sometimes I think that I am losing

You are soft
Tho you do not give in
You are tough
Yet you think that love is a sin
I am speaking of love with me
You should not for you know of my history
If you know not by now then you should
Because my love is good
Just look at what I am doing now
Trying to write of love yet I do not know how
Sometimes I think that I am losing
Often my heart is bruising
Over how may I stay in touch
Without causing you such
Trouble
Then I back off upon the double
Tho I do not want to be alone
I would like to talk on the phone
I just have to speak face to face
Tho I well know that we shall move at your pace
I will not go ahead for I shall wait
Because true love will not be late
Leigh knows that I love Leigh
I love all of her and she
Loves for me to love her
There is not a need for her to call me sir
Nor for me to call her lady
Because with love we are going steady.

LETTERS TO LEIGH

My heart is on the pyre

You might think that I am being lazy
All of my thoughts are kind of hazy
 my feelings seem kind of crazy
Yet my tender love for you is kind of easy
I cannot escape that fact
Even if I use all of my tact
I shall still always know
That only with you I will be whole
I need to talk to you badly
For now I wish that I had, sadly,
A way of changing things
of hearing you sing
For of your sound I could never tire
You know that I am not a liar
My heart is on the pyre
It is up to you to start the fire
the only thing that will put it out
Is for you to open up your love fount
I wish that I could plainly make my case
When next we meet face to face
Yet now I have a fear
That I will not see you this year
Now I feel my heart tear
As I feel my teardrops sear
Across my face
That slowly trace
From my eyes
To where my heart sighs.

LETTERS TO LEIGH

When we are home

I know that each passing day
Only makes you delay
Yet I know there is a way
On calling on love to stay
Love that I have known
that seems to have flown
Back to its nest
Which is us being alone
With the love that was sown
When we first met
for if love we let
Take that slow, kind course
We shall find that it pours
Down from above
Upon us, little dove
We shall soak it up
then drink from loves cup
We will take our bath
In love then we shall laugh
Because the best
Is the love fest
To come
When we are home
I will love you always
I shall kneel then I will pray
Giving thanks above,
Thank thee for this special love

LETTERS TO LEIGH

I am going to sound loves bugle call

Love is something hard to measure
We search for it as if it was lost and buried
treasure
Love for you is not hard to pronounce
When you show your love on it I will pounce
I am thinking that I am playing with fire
Of that I shall never tire
For your love is like hot coals
Am I able to handle it, you should know
Let me put my arms around your waist
Allow your tongue to my lips taste
Hold me while I place one hand in your hair
As the other does pull you near
May I kiss your eyebrows
Ever let me wonder how
That I could have such luck
To have you then your palms to suck
Please excuse me if I am blunt
For I have been a long time on the hunt
I am hungry for love like a wolf
Of your love I shall soon be stuffed
From draughting in that love my thirst will be
quenched
Upon your love I shall soon be lynched
Only you may untie the knot
 I will be hoping that you forgot
I am going to sound loves bugle call
We shall find out if my love will fall
 will I not be there to catch your frown
Even if love knocked you down.

LETTERS TO LEIGH

To leave you with a tear stain in your eyes

I love you Leigh
That is my problem
To hear from you
Would be love balm on
All of my pain
To do thus would be a cane
To my heart that is sprained
Which is the same
As my soul which is stained
Our love cannot be blamed
I am to blame for leaving
Thus leaving you grieving
I am at fault
Twas kind of an insult
To leave you with a tear stain in your eyes
With only a guilty good-bye
I still remember your reply
When finally I answered I did not lie
Did I not say, I love you, too,
What I said was true
I want to be your fool
Your love pool
There I would mount
Your love fount
Then whenever you like
I may unplug the dike
Letting love flood
Wheresoever that it should.

LETTERS TO LEIGH

By your own choice

Maybe you will not call
Perhaps my heart shall fall
Maybe I will just say
That I love you anyway
I cannot see what is going on
At that home
Where you are all alone
Beside the phone
Go ahead and pick it up
Slowly then it let your hands cup
Raise it to your lips and sup
Then look down and let it drop
Until you are ready
To hold it steady
Do not be shy
Because you may rely
That I will hang on
If you shall be strong
You know that I am waiting
While anticipating
Having the pleasure
Beyond all measure
Of hearing your voice
By your own choice
If you choose to sing
Make the phone go ring-a-ling
Just pick up the phone
Then let your love roam.

LETTERS TO LEIGH

Yet my favourite way

I may have time for stress after awhile
right now all I have to do is smile
keep it down low
Where it does not show
 I may take a walk
Or have a talk
With a friend of mine
If they have the time
 if they do not
I shall haunt
All of this stress
That is importantly dressed
Right out of my body
While I go on with my hobby
Or maybe I shall go into a deep
Thought sleep
Then I will daydream
On the banks of a stream
For with all of my luck
Stress I shall have struck
Yet my favourite way
Is at the end of the day
When I think of you
Of the love due,
Just some thoughts
Of you whom I have sought
Now I may lay down
Without even a frown.

LETTERS TO LEIGH

Watching the wind blow

Watching the grass grow
Watching the wind blow
Waiting on a leaf to fall
Waiting on you to call
All do take some time
For all are sublime,
My patience I hold dear
Your love I ever hold near
As I await from you to hear
My heart begins to slowly tear
My Leigh, my Leigh, my Leigh, my Leigh
I still feel that you are a part of me
Have not I already paid loves fee
I am begging you on bended knee
In sleep you call my name
Awake you may do the same
My heart is intended for you to tame
Tho it is not meant for you to maim
It is not a mistake that I have made
For all of loves fees I have not paid
Yet all of my heart down I have laid
Take it before it does turn to jade
I shall pay love with these drops
As I have hope that from me love soon will hop
From me to you until it must fill your heart to the
top
Then into your soul it finally does stop
Where it will open the door
For to let your love come forth.

LETTERS TO LEIGH

Then we will have not more good-byes

My love still does not hurt yet
Yet as for yours, I would not bet
Does your love feel good and let
Your heart know that in love it is set
do you feel all blue
With a feeling like you are being used
In some way that I cannot name
By a love that you may not ever tame
I think that you may feel shame
Then maybe think that I will take the blame
Shall I accept it, you know that I will
Of your love I shall drink my fill
It is your love that I would love to fulfil
I will keep hoping that to become so until
You stop and turn around
When my love you have found
As you have hearkened to my sound
Then with my love you are bound
To take me to paradise
Just by looking in your eyes
There I shall listen to your sighs
Then we will have not more good-byes
I love you Leigh, as I have said before
Even if my love you do ignore
Do not leave my heart scarred and torn
Leave it with the eagles to forever soar
My cast of love for you is not a gamble
If I win you, all of the woman that I need ever
handle.

LETTERS TO LEIGH

Do you think, after all,

She might call me today
She may want to say
That her love due s she will pay
If my love down I will lay
I really love you Leigh
Come to me then stay
I want to hold you tight
Through your darkest night
I would like to be your light
So that you may have sight
For if we continue on this trend
Our hearts will make amends
We shall be better friends
Then our hearts will each other send
Us on a love binge
As all of our love shall hinge
On how often our love will singe
then how far love shall infringe
On all of our lesser emotions
So let us apply love potion
then if you take the notion
add to that love lotion
We will be nice and slick
As your lips I lick
I shall think of other tricks
Do you think, after all,
That you should call.

LETTERS TO LEIGH

Just take me away to then

I am still wishing that it was April
When I had those hands to feel
I thought that it was a good deal
When your kisses I used to steal
I knew that you were please inside
Even if that you tried to hide
It was hard, for your blush died
Your smile and that never lied
Just take me away to then
When we were such good friends
Give back to me the time when
Your heart you often used to lend
I shall take time to linger
To place a ring upon your finger
To make of you a singer
to remove from you the stinger
That he left inside of your breast
To take the poison from you lest
It does spread then the rest
Of it becomes a cruel jest
Just move your hand
I will suck the poison out
Allow me to wave my wand
So that the poison becomes a love fount
It is you that I want to heal
you that I want to feel
My heart you may peel
Yours I only want to steal.

LETTERS TO LEIGH

Love together we will share

I wish that you were coming soon
We would stay up and watch the moon
Making love until noon
With our hearts strewn
All about
An open fount
With love seeping out
Where love would mount
To ride beside
The rising of the tide
Without reason to hide
There I will bide
Riding the gentle swells
Of where I rose then where I fell
Only time may tell
If this is a gentle hell
Our sins it may dispel
Then lead us unto an angel
More than anything else in the world
I want our love to fly unfurled
We shall one day plant it on a grassy knurl
We will be under it in arms curled
because I love you I think that we should
Come together any way that we could
Talk to each other any way that we would
Walk that way each step that we trod
Hearts together we shall get there
Love together we will share.

Love to make your heart mend

You are like something that I crave
Something that has been saved
With good intentions paved
For me to leave my cave
I will come on out
Shall I not turn about
While I give a shout
Then have a pout
If you are not there
To meet my stare
Then like a bear
I will return to my lair
Yet I shall leave the door open
 I will turn to look when
You have started to wend
Toward me then I would send
Love to make your heart mend
For that would lead you to tend
To offer friendship then lend
love on me and I would spend
Your love money
All of your love honey,
It will not be funny
When you are my bunny
I shall give you treats
In the form of heat
I will give you love
Like from above.

LETTERS TO LEIGH

Let love come to the fore

I do not feel like writing tonight
My feelings do make my hands move a slight
I stop for a smoke to light
then my heart catches sight
Of your love shining bright
So that I put up the fight
By taking time to write
That- that your heart bites
I have never been so sincere
As when I held you near
Your heart would never sear
As when I held you, dear
Our last meeting
Was just the beginning
Soon we will be greeting
then we shall be pinning
Each other with rings
For we will sing
About love then any odd thing
Until happiness does bring
To us a fine spirit
We shall be willing to share it
We will not ever have reason to fear it
Our feeling, will we bare it
I could say that I wish more
For I have more words in store
Yet I would not want to bore
Let love come to the fore.

LETTERS TO LEIGH

Inside of your heart

I would like to have this poem written
Because by love I have been bitten
By your charms I have been smitten
I love you and I am not quitting
I find that it is only fitting
That in love we are sitting
Please do not say that you do not think so
For when I have you then you shall know
For what you will do
Knowing again how loves feeling does feel so..
I know that you will help some
To know love you will come
Into your loves home
You shall know where love is from
To know how it does start
Inside of your heart
You will know which part
When it does feel loves dart
Then like a sweet tart
Soon does depart
Yet it always must leave a grin
Which does begin
With its only wile
To soon become a smile
I shall kiss you then
You will know when
In my eyes you are my prize.

LETTERS TO LEIGH

Live, let us, again

I am doing things that I think I should not
I know that if I had you I could not
I do not like it much myself
For losing you is bad for my health
I am in a wrong way walking with stealth
Too much I think of acquiring wealth
Happiness, my happiness, is leaving
As for the want of you, the more I am grieving
While your love I am bereaving
Am I my mind deceiving
Now my heart is heaving
As I am my soul leaving
Are you my wits peeving
My love you are only thieving
Surely you do not
Have to do that sad task
Just come lift me off of this lonely cot
Then pour slowly from true loves flask
To me then come save from my sad habit
For a broken heart that is in need of healing must
share it
Now far above the silent din
Your eyes seem full of hope, yes they are open
For love let me look there-in
May my refection seek not sin
Live, let us, again
As one
Has that which was lost been won,
shall we taste once more loves simple balm.

.

LETTERS TO LEIGH

Whisper sweet words into your ear

You may have thought that it was all a game
Yet I did fall in love all of the same
Your falling for me was my aim
I did not want for it to be a game
Maybe that was my sin
If twas, I would do it all again
Only next time should I not play to win
I would tear up the rule book then
Whisper sweet words into your ear
Words that only you could hear
That should then put our love into gear
We could fall in love with nothing to fear
As I kiss you on the lips
From your love I would take a sip
For you my heart should flip
Over me your heart would skip
I should have you all for myself
Making love until only love is left
I could kiss where your breast cleft
Then lower my kisses slowly by stealth
I should take a double handful
Being careful not to soil
What recompense for all of my toil
Only our blood to boil
I would love you from smallest toe
To your hairdo
Then I could begin to woo.

LETTERS TO LEIGH

You I love so much

With love pressing close, I am walking about
From my ending toes
Toward my slanting nose
Walk I for you and pose
To you I love so much
Want I only to touch
Should only I, only I hold you
Just love making will not do
Some money today found I in the mail
Felt I that the sensation was quite stale
Wouldst that love was for sale
Should I then tell
That of hers I so want, pledge I to her many
Then cast down my last penny
Want she ask of any
Ask she I hope for tenny
Give all to her I have
have I all of that saved
Should I lay it into her hand
Filling like a man
Would I go from there
To above where
love lays upstairs
In its upstairs lair
Her love could I take all at once
Would I on it pounce
Should all my money I flounce
All of my love pence.

LETTERS TO LEIGH

When we feel loves dart

Wouldst me let love until you tired
Shouldst then give I what you desired
Until on you were afire
Just a prior
To a way of finding out
Happily with a shout
then would love sprout
Out from crying love fount
Finally where we there mount
Shall we finally have a taste
Never will shall waste
Nor maketh haste
As the other each baste
With love lotion
 a sweet potion
Gently with motion
To us come shall a solution
As to whether we are together when apart
then just close our minds to start
Follow we into one heart
When feel we loves dart
Be I yours
Shall you be mine
Through the hours
Ending time
Are you love
or of treasure a lonesome trove.

LETTERS TO LEIGH

That you might so live

Afraid not am I to ask
To do loves task
Because I do not want
To hear you say no
Want do I not that it be known
That your frown
Shown
Should fuse of love not be blown
You this heart do rend
A way must find it to mend
Before it can send
To you love to lend
Must I this heart then bare
Am I your love to share
All that I offer I give
That you might so live
In what you offer of return
All take it I then learn
With that loves sweet taste
Shall make we a sweet paste
Will we with haste
To our hearts baste
Before they burn
Take shall we a turn
At the fire
Of desire
Will we then mount
To it put out.

LETTERS TO LEIGH

Hoping that love will start

This is the last page
The last act of love on the stage
Love will set the wage
Then my love shall rage
Me on to play my part
Hoping that love will start
To grow inside of your heart
For into that I shall place loves dart
Until I touch that special spot
With a lot
Of love that is red hot
Right onto the dot
Of where you may need love the most
To your love I shall be host
I do not want your feelings to roast
Nor do I wish for me to boast
I need only for my love toward you to count
Then my love for you to fount
As your soul I do plan to haunt
For yours does mine then constantly taunts
Me on to more
Until with you I reach loves shores
There I will love your heart that is sore
As you shall love mine that you tore
We will live as man and wife
For we shall have each other for life
Then we may look back on yesterday
As when we let our love play.

LETTERS TO LEIGH

When you are all alone

Fantasy is artificial
Love is real
For once would I like to feel
This broken heart heal
I think that we should seal
That with a kiss and deal
With falling for one another
We are no longer sister and brother
I cannot be your friend
Because our love we send
Back and forth again
Lovers we want to be
Do not you want to see
You are all that I want in life
Come, please be my wife
Maybe one of these nights
To you shall come the light
When you are all alone
You will see that I am the one
Who may ease the pain
Then delay the rain
To fall only upon your garden
Then love may grant a pardon
I want to save you for myself
Should I not have all of your love that is left
When I have it
Then we may sit
As together our hearts knit.

LETTERS TO LEIGH

There I shall stay

Should pain feel good
When it does end
Pleasure should
Make amends
All of the sorrow
Will not be tomorrow
Shall there be any to borrow
Or only love to follow
Will we drink our fill
As I kneel
At your feet
To kiss so sweet
Those knees
Should I beg, please,
Allow me to try
Ascendingly high
While my lips rise
Up to your thigh
Will I give a sigh
As back you shall lie
Will you take your rest
Hand upon breast
Shall I take that then
Letting go when
You let it slip
As you moisten lips
That I put the fire into your desire
There I shall stay if you like it that way.

LETTERS TO LEIGH

Like a nest

After many stale years
All that is left is your stare
With my eyes full of tears
You took all that I had
I found more
You have made my heart sad
Then left it so sore
I am thinking of you now
Just sitting here thinking
I am wondering how
Because my heart is still blinking
It may take a year
For me to forget
With many a tear
Then heartbreak yet
Like a nest
Up in a tree
I am holding on lest
You fall away from me
I am also like the ground
Should you happen to fall
I will hear your sound
Then catch eggs and all
I would gently take my hand
To lift them up
Out of the sand
Into loves cup.

LETTERS TO LEIGH

We may spread our love around

I am the arrow
You are the bow
You I will deliver
With our quiver
You are the lock
I am the key
That shall release the stocks
Setting your free
You are like a cat
So slick
I am the rat
Involved in your trick
I am kind of tired from playing cat and mouse
Let us just quit to set up house
We may spread our love around
With all of its sweet, sweet sound
Let us just drift along with the breeze
Making love beneath the trees
Then as we stop to have a drink
Shall we not drive love to the brink
As far as love will go
Who does know
What blessing
May be in store
While we are messing
With more
Love coming
As love is foaming.

Would you care for more?

I may find another
Way to smother
You with affection
Then if there is rejection
I shall find another way
For your love to sway
For winning is why I play
Anything I will say
Hurry, do not delay
Take my heart upon a tray
Unto your fire
Where with your desire
You may make it roast
Playfully then boast
 it you may then taste
While with love baste
You may broil
Even stab it with your foil
When it is nice and tender
Before this feeling is all a cinder
You may have a feast
Upon my love which is the least
That I can do
While I woo
You so gently
I simply
Have to know the score
Would you care for more.

LETTERS TO LEIGH

To make you whole

Does anyone know
How deep my love should go
With stealth
Let us try the depth
I will go first
Because I have a thirst
For you to come
Try the foam
If you like it
Come in and sit
As the waves do rise
Around your thighs
Lay back and drift
Let love sift
Through that feeling
That you should feel sealing
Upon your heart
Then let it start
To make you whole
Heart and soul
 yes feel my love
Begin to prove
That it is safe swimming
As long as you are hemming
It in with your being
Are you now seeing
You will stay ever young
While singing loves song.

LETTERS TO LEIGH

Let us let love be

What was then true yesterday
Is so today
I do want it to be shown
That your love I alone own
I would like for all to know
What true love may sow
That we may reap
Our love to keep
I need to look into your stare
Then know that our love is rare
For our love is fair
With both of our hearts laid so bare
Should not our love be effective
Of the best to be selective
If I had to choose
I would offer my heart to use
Even if I lose
If it be so, abused
Oh, I do love you
That is so true
With you I want to go
All with you I want to do
Just come along
Sing your song
Love me
You will see
That I love thee
Let us let love be.

LETTERS TO LEIGH

You say, be a friend

You are the most extraordinarily
Beautiful woman when you cry....
Yet I
Do even want to see you sigh
When you giggle
My love does wiggle
I have to keep going
With love flowing
As love is sowing
Tho a favourite of mine
Is when you are crying
Except for when
You say, be a friend,
That is when I say,
Love shall find a way,
Then you nod
Saying, if it is the will of God,
I shall agree
Then together we
Try to be friends
Oddly, tho, there is not an end
Of our love going
To each and showing
That we belong
Like your song
That never did wrong.
Which goes on alone

LETTERS TO LEIGH

So that your love is bare

You see me writing in this love book
Are you able to tell how much love that it has took
It is waiting in a nook
If you should like to take a look
Just take my heart
Then open it in part
Hold, do not start
To push loves dart
Too, too deep
For being made
To wade
May slow you down
Let it become so that if you drown
In love
My own will shove
You up toward the air
So that your love is bare
Until your stare
Is shining fair
There you may say you have waited
With breath abated
Until we have in our hands
Each ones love wands
Then, if taken by the notion,
Shaken love potion.

.

LETTERS TO LEIGH

Softly, I have a friend

I have two hands
In each
Hold I two wands
With which I teach
My wand is my pen
Unlike other men
Gold I do not hoard
Nor shall I take you by sword
With my pen I try
To make you smile and cry
For I always win
When you grin
That does tell me again
Softly, I have a friend
Tho if you shed a tear
May I take it so to smear
A liquid pearl into my ink
Then into that sink
For you are my link
With heaven
I am not leaving
You to face the heathen
While I am breathing
For I shall be hard trying
To keep you from sighing
Then if you begin crying
I will swallow my lying
Then follow with my heart dying.

LETTERS TO LEIGH

I will bring you joy

Every time that you send me away
In your hand a piece of me does stay
When you notice will you it lay
In a safe place for me, until another day
For you I am on my knees
Asking of God, please,
Let love squeeze
From thee her hearts keys,
I would take that ring
For you I should then sing
Until you would bring
Love fit for a king
On that I would dine
With loves fine
Wine
Would I not eat like a lion
All of the night long
Until birdsong awoke
At the time that you spoke
Without wrong
Only just to sing along
I will bring you joy
You shall say, o-boy!,
As I start to slumber
I will pull you under
The quilt
That our love built.

LETTERS TO LEIGH

Have not fear

Love is full of questions
Mine does seem to be full of confessions
For instance,
Am I taking a chance
On loving you
That while I am wooing
My love is yet proving
That love is good
Just as it should
For it is going along
With your song
Tho you are there
While I am where
Still I may sing
Holding your ring
With me yet is your necklace
Right beneath my face
I have your photo
Laid aside for now
I shall take care
That it does not tear
Have not fear,
I am here
To touch your hair
Then catch a falling tear
Could I not match that one
With all that I own.

LETTERS TO LEIGH

If I only had the treasure

If I had treasure up above
Would I not send a prayer upward like a dove
Should I not ask for permission
To call for an intermission
Asking for him to lend
For him to send
Loves legal tender so that I may send her
Into the way
Where love does lay
If I had treasure down below
Would I not take it then stow
All into a chest
Then at your behest
Should I not pay your cost
Before you became lost
Would I not give my last penny
Before I lost you any
If I had treasure in my hand
Should I not throw it down to the sand
Then fill my palm
With your love balm
Then rub it around
While hearing that sweet sound
 so close to be found
If I had only the treasure
That would bring you pleasure.

Love is not fair

If you like what I do send
More love have I to lend
Through the clouds up above
Send I to thee my pure love
Upon the wings of a dove
Send I these thoughts that may be wove
Into a clear garment
To end the daily torment
For a little while
Then cause me to smile
While of you thinking
Of when you were blinking
Am I into love sinking
As I picture you winking
Love is not fair
To separate and tear
You and I apart
When love had just begun to start
To touch our heart
Within the part
That feels the dart
Could that tell us that love does glow
A silent flame
To let us know
We are not of shame
Into love we have came
 even the same.

LETTERS TO LEIGH

Until I fell

Out of love does bloom
A rose
May out of love loom
My nose
Near enough
To smell,
To touch
Then I fell
Into her bloom
There was room
For me to stay
To play
Loved I the smell
For climbed I to the top
Until I fell
Then upon a thorn did stop
Hang I onto my thorn
Twas I not forlorn
For this too I did know
Was a part of my rose
As I sat I would talk
To the stalk
Said I, tell the rose
If it happened to know
That the seed that love does sow
Is here to show,
For her to dip that delicate flower
To let love on me then shower.

Like fine wine

The heart as a muscle
Does flex
When trying to rustle
One of the opposite sex
Inside of each eye
Is fine wine
In them without lie
Is a vintage so fine
As a rose
Your nose
Does pose
As a dimply show
Poise
Like a toy
Placed
Upon your face
A gentle trace
As of delicate lace
May I kiss a lip
From there take a sip
to my way up
Towered the bottom of the cup
Then
Fill again
Then hold
Until you are bold
When silence becomes willing
To keep on filling.

LETTERS TO LEIGH

Around my heart

Have I found my love cup
Yet still need loves spoon
To stir it up
I hope to find it soon
All of the sugar
Is on the bottom
The creamer
Is still floating
Is it too hot
To sip
Will I not
Burn my lip
Shall I wait awhile
Upon my face a smile
Watching this love pool
Waiting on loves tool
Now and then
Will I hold it up
Shall I know when
To sup
Would I drink it slow
Allowing love to flow
Around my heart
Which will start
To take the pain
Out of my brain
To help my soul
Become whole.

LETTERS TO LEIGH

Will I maintain faith

Would I ever tear
My love
Would I share
Not shove
Am I an optimist
Do I want not to be a pest
Have you told me that you love me before
Shall you think that you I ignore
Words that you have shown
Soft sayings you do own
Will I maintain faith
Upon your hearts lathe
My love does turn
As that lonely heart does burn
Shall I ever forget
I promise I will not
You shall not me let
For you are a constant thought
Constantly you tease
Write I to appease
Have you engaged an eye
Are you a constant sigh
That I ex-hale
When my life does feel stale
Am I your life buoy
Although I may annoy
May I not save
From of love a wave.

LETTERS TO LEIGH

You will not lay me down

Myself you may need
To read
A romantic encyclopaedia
Of love a cornucopia
If me you do pick up
You will not lay me down
My love shall you sup
On my love that has shown
thru and over constant day
In many a way
you will not lay me down
Nor may disown
For to your ear
There are silent sweet words to hear
Within your lip
Such love to sip
For to smell
An ambrosian shell
Such
A feeling to touch
In each eye
Not a lie
For your hair
Have my stare
Drink deep of all and still
There is more so have your fill
While there is a failing light
May pleasure come falling upon your night.

LETTERS TO LEIGH

Shall we have not choice

Is my love real
Would I your love steal
Should your heart peel
Unto my loves will
 are you acting haughty
Shall I be acting naughty
By committing a theft
Of your heart with stealth
When all is said then done
Will we say that love has won
Shall we have not a choice
Only to rejoice
Will I pay you recompense
In this instance
With all of the love that I carry
Then if you do want to marry
Shall you have love to keep
Will my love you reap,
The harvest of my heart
May be taken into your mart
Then rub and make it shine
Was ever love so fine
Shall I drink your love like wine
Then with that dine
Upon loves feast
Until I have the breast
Over the heart which lies inside
Of you my bride.

LETTERS TO LEIGH

That all of your love is not showing

Is your heart a fountain
On top o loves mountain
If I may have a taste
Promise I not to waste
Give me if you may a drop
Will I ever stop from keeping
The fount weeping
Shall I listen unto my own word
One that will prick love as a sword
Until drop by drop I then drink
While as doing more of those ways so think
 I to keep your love flowing
If even I am knowing
That all of your love is not showing
What I may, I will gather
Shall I not your love tether
Will I let it flow
 as to take love in slow
Shall I take love in a way that is fast
While it does last
Should that be the case
Will I be the vase
Into which may your love follow
That even more love does swallow
If ever I make the fount fair
Where
Your love shall you share.

LETTERS TO LEIGH

We must make two, one heart,

What is the cost
Of our love
That we lost
How do we account
For such an amount
How should we figure
Then measure
Our loss so tremendous
A cost so stupendous
Half of our love is in me
The other half is in thee
To have our love back into one part
We must make two, one heart,
Our heart torn, each others halve
Should be healed by love salve
Our love may be made strong
To stay away from what went wrong
Our heart may sound loves song
From morning all of the day long
You have the lock
Holding love inside the dungeon of rock
I must find the key
Then shall we
Be one
A total fraction
Of satisfaction
From the interest drawn
For having in love fallen.

LETTERS TO LEIGH

Then from there take a sip

Am I taking off this necklace
Do I feel reckless
Has it left a scar
Where your lips once were
Now hold it I in my hand
In the other hold I my wand
Do I intend to write in this way
Am I hoping for your love to sway
Is it still my love charm
Want I to keep it from harm
As I cherish you shall I cherish it
Also the ring to make sure it does fit
Will I lay it with your love letter
Shall maybe then it make me feel better
Then if my eyes even grow wetter
From being bound into loves fetter
Will I place it upon my lip
Then from there take a sip
Finally I am done
When having then found myself all alone
Shall I put it on
For the thoughts your love have sown
Those that keep my heart
From becoming stone
Shall I then start
One by lonely one
To fold each page
Wherein love does dance about the stage.

LETTERS TO LEIGH

My soul it is that you soothe

There are many things that I may live without
Kind of sadly, that does not include my love fount
I am working up a powerful thirst
When I do drink, I may burst
Of taking a long draught
From my love fount
Quite a waterfall
On her love I shall call
While standing underneath
That watery sheath
Then maybe stroll
Into loves pool
Where taking a dip
Love I sip
Drinking all
Yet not full
Maybe I would then play
Inside of the spray
With a mute kiss
Toward the silent mist
I hold onto this water hole
Like I do my soul
To tell all of the truth
My soul it is that you soothe
In case you may not know
I am in love with you
Let us not speak in jest
We are ready for loves test.

LETTERS TO LEIGH

Having not spite, nor hate

Are you having a good day
May I tell from the way
That I feel, and say
Would you, I bet, like to play
Because I would
Do you not think that you should
Feel great
Having not spite, nor hate
Is love within the air
Does it not feel fair
Am I hoping for you the best
Every day a fest
With never a distraction
Only to have pure satisfaction
Wish I you well in life
Have not disturbance nor strife
Only to live on easy street
Shoes so new upon your feet
May a breeze be about your face
While dressed all over with delicate lace
Do I hope your roof does not leak
Hope I that you have not clothes with holes that
peek
Please have good things to eat
With pleasant friends to greet
May I help not to let this slip in,
Although it may be a sin,
Oh, just use your imagination
So as to finish the equation

LETTERS TO LEIGH

From the heart

I do not feel
That you could not steal
This loving word
Or disturb
Me if I did not want you
To
Yet I do
So
Keep on
Taking each poem
Throw them down
Where they will not be found
I shall write more
For you to ignore
Because the more that you read
You so bleed
From the heart
Where love did start
You are not hurting
Me
Yet my heart is smarting,
Leigh
One day closely does follow
Another then that one did swallow
What went before
So do not be sore
Tho if you are
I have the cure.

LETTERS TO LEIGH

Down to the end

Are we alike
Have we precious impulses in Gods sight
Those that go unfulfilled
Make the troubled waters still
Good intentions count more
That do deeds when the heart is sore
I am able to know that your heart is soft
From your wet eyes and your cough
When you thought that badly I was feeling
As I to you was kneeling
I handled it with a grin
Then yours came back again
I never liked to see your tear
Nor ever liked to see you cry
I somehow helped ease your fear
Somehow then dried your eye
That you were crying for me I know
I just did not let my tear show
Calmly I took bad news
Then made so much look like few
In the state that we were in
If I had it all to do again
I would not know if I could otherwise do
Or even differently woo
Because we were one another's friend
Down to the end
Even if I could
I do not know if I should.

LETTERS TO LEIGH

Like a sweet tart

Have I my favourite cigar
I have my only drink
As I am writing to my sugar
Into love I do now sink
In a blink
Of an eye
You shall sink
With a sigh
Sexy music
On the radio
Only does stick
Up my libido
I pick my cigar
Up
Then I write to my sugar
While I drink from my cup
The taste
Does depart
With haste
Like a sweet tart
I am in remiss
It is like your kiss
Now this pen
That I hold
Has a yen
To be bold
Until it does slip
Against that retreating lip.

Always nice to me

I cannot get you out of my mind
I look around then it is you that I find
You could say
That it is sweet misery
 you might say
Surely this is sweet hell to play
With your hallucination
Inside of my imagination
Any way that you say it
You should know that I do love it
It is kind of convenient
Because you are quite lenient
For to have you around
Just to hear your sound
Then you I take along
To hear you sing your song
There it is with ease
That I find you to please
I may make you grin
When I call you friend
You are pleasant company
Always nice to me
I will love you forever
Trying not to sever
This thing
That you bring
Your face
Inside of my hearts place.

LETTERS TO LEIGH

Begging you to bring your tear

Someday I hope for you to read this
I hope for you to feel some bliss
Knowing that I loved you so
Ever have I continued to woo
While you were far away
Where you so long had to stay
Yet if you are reading this it is known
That from that place you have flown
You have found me with open arms
To escape from the following storms
You always knew that I was here
Begging you to bring your tear
I knew how to end your fear
You have a new life
Now that you have left that lonely bier
I have saved some money
To help you feel like a honey
You just may have fled
Into my bed
Leaving the strife
To become my wife
To you I will not say no
Oh God, let it be so
You are all that I want in life
I will not lose you like a knife
Let me love you please
I am already on my knees
Please come soon
Be here maybe by noon.

LETTERS TO LEIGH

About my hearts incision

I still have it inside of my head
That you love me instead
You planted that seed
To you that may be as a weed
Tho I think what you have sown
Has taken on wings then flown
From off of the floor
Up to soar
High above
Common love
There it does wait
At steady gait
As it does grow
Love begins to flow
Into that vein
To replace each stain
Of the past
That does last
Yet what I do need you
To know
Is that I shall do all
To soften your fall
I will swoop down
To ease your frown
May I place over you a shade
Until you have made
That little decision
About my hearts incision.

LETTERS TO LEIGH

From my soap bubble

I cannot think when I think of you
I only blink
Then wince
Finding that out as I give myself a pinch
Why did I not cry
I dared not lie
Did not I try
For you to fly
Anything then I could have done
That I may have won
I want for you a baby
Not to have a hysterectomy
Your baby would be my portion
Not for you an abortion
That could bring a curse for
What we would rehearse so poor
May I lose my right arm
Before you suffer harm
Let me have my evil nightmare
Before you see worse care
There is not a doubt
That I would have a bout
With trouble
Before a pout
Upon my soap bubble
Who I would hold in this hand
As I do my wand
Then place atop of loves pond.

LETTERS TO LEIGH

Always doing something good

It is common for us to have a delusion
Tho mine of you does give an infusion
Into that vein
Which is not to blame
For carrying love
Up above
To my brain
Which does become lame
Without the power
That your love does shower
Onto my physique
It is all mystique
How does it this
That is
Always doing something good
Like we should
The collateral benefit
Is that my mind will not quit
Until it has found
The source of the sound
That does play inside of my ear
Which I constantly hear
I think that back I shall trace
 right to your face
All the while that I have been flying
You may have been crying
Shall I take your tear
Then into mine smear.

LETTERS TO LEIGH

Trying to not do anything wrong

All that I need is a miracle
Even one that is partial
I am watching myself all day long
Trying to not do anything wrong
I must seek to be on Gods good side
 only he may turn the tide
If he did still talk to men
I would ask for him to send
To you an angel
For all of your reasons to mangle
May he give to you new sight
Then you shall see the light
That when time was planned
We were meant as man and woman
I am willing to wait ten years
Saving all of my tears
All that I want is you
Thoughts of others have flew
When we met
You and I let
Our emotion
Give us the solution
Therefore do not be afraid
If your love for him is dead
I shall love you more
If you are knocked down to the floor
Yet I hope that does not happen
As our love I am mapping.

LETTERS TO LEIGH

As love does churn

The least that I may do
If I cannot write
Is to think of you
As your light
You shed all around
Wherever you are found
Here I make it to be my aim
To come near unto your flame
That I intend to tame
Until we are the same
Height
In each others sight
I shall take you as a candle
Hold you then by the handle
Light you at each end
Until your middle does unbend
Then like hot wax
You may relax
Here by my side
Then take a ride
Where love does rule
For we are only of love a tool
When you are in the mood
May I never be rude
For we each shall learn
As love does churn
All, it would seem
blending the finest of sugar and crème.

LETTERS TO LEIGH

You have turned me inside out

I had rather be with you in this way
Than to be with others and to play
You are my hope with my dream
It is you who does fill me full of steam
You have made me clean
Your love machine
That healing voice
Overcame all of the noise
That gentle lip
Gave unto me love to sip
That nature alone
Touched me to the bone
Through the haze
I await that gaze
That beautiful laughter
Does raise my temperature
Yet when I have a fever
You always find the lever
To bring it down
Changing my frown
With all of my bile
Into a grin
To love again
You have turned me inside out
My long sought for love fount
You I do love to stroke and pet
Tell me, do you feel love yet.

LETTERS TO LEIGH

For this reason it is that I live

May one day my prayer make it through
Then he your heart could move
All of my feeling I would prove
That this heart talk for you is true
With this intent
Do I bare my heart to be rent
Love for you I have not all spent
Only to you I have lent
May you have all that I do give
For this reason it is that I live
With me there is nothing to forgive
As I seek a thought of you I am all a-quiv
I know that there is a way
A coming day
That we shall say hello
Then that will swallow
All of the past
To forever last
That long
With our song
When
I take my pen
To immortalize
Then tantalize
With a sigh
While eye to eye
As I see you again
That will be worth all that has been.

LETTERS TO LEIGH

I would feel the same way

As you walked across the floor
Did you almost stop at the door
Then turn enough around
For me to see your frown
I saw enough to ably tell
That you were in a living hell
Because having to choose
Left a sore bruise
Because I could almost see
Your heart bleed
I knew that it was a tough choice
Without cause to rejoice
You so missed your little boy
The touch of his voice
I would feel the same way
Yet I could not leave you, Leigh
Not the other self
That I need for my health
Then as you stood at the door
I could not ignore
Your posture
That you did foster
For my benefit
Yet I did see through it
During this moment
I saw your torment
Then I did know
You do love me so.

LETTERS TO LEIGH

I tell you that every day

I may not ever get over you Leigh
I hope that it is not just me
I may only do my best
As I wait on love to do the rest
What more do I have to say
That down my love I do lay
I tell you that every day
While all of the time I do pray
For you to love me again
If not that, only to me stay a friend
Both or one will do
While I find a way to woo
From your hair above to shoe down low
Even more than I used to
I shall ever know that you are a lady
While claiming every baby
I could not yours ignore
Playing upon the floor
Then up into love we soar
Ready to make more
After time has had enough
Toward one another never tough
We place aside our thoughts cuff
As we talk of other stuff
I shall have not hesitation
In making conversation
Because the way that we are conversing
Requires little rehearsing.

LETTERS TO LEIGH

You make me so happy

Happiness is like a pill
That I shall take until
I have had my fill
While my senses do reel
It has a pleasant taste
None will I waste
It is best going down
When you have a frown
Until sadness drowns
Into happiness thrown
If pure happiness came in a bottle
With it I would ever cuddle
Then take it as a drug
Without a shrug
Yet I do not have to hope
That happiness was like dope
Tho I am alone
You still hold my funny-bone
When you give it a wiggle
I start to giggle
As thoughts of you
Turn my black skies blue
For you do make me so happy
I am talking about you, Leigh
I ever have you with me
In my memory
I do not want it to be past
While the pain does last.

LETTERS TO LEIGH

I just told the truth

God the serpent cursed
For the lie that it rehearsed
I now draw on him
As I sit on a limb
Ready to strike
It in the neck
For tempting me
To lie to Leigh
Yet I am glad
That her trust I had
It I have kept
While she has slept
Her soft hearts snore
Is becoming less easy to ignore
I could not find a way to soothe
I just told the truth
About my situation
Without hesitation
Then her participation
Was a taste of heaven
To my way of looking
Her love I was booking
I had to start
In the best part
With the someone
That I did not have to fool
For she was loves willing tool.

LETTERS TO LEIGH

Within the sunshine

May my faith move the mountain
In which flows my waterfall
I may find my fountain
With love standing tall
These words may be special
That must depend on how you feel
I know Thai I have one feeling, surely it I feel
It is this, my heart at your feet does kneel
 I would like to make it nice and plain
That to you my love I am paying
This emotion may clean my stain
Please pay attention to what I am saying
I may not be sophisticated
Nor in love well educated
Yet at least give me credit
While you have taken your love and hid it
I will be waiting near heavens gate
Inviting you to participate
I beg you not to wait
Love cannot be too late
I want to greet you as a friend
Then have with you time to spend
That shall be a day
To come on out and play
Within the sunshine
In loves clime
Since we are near there
I will add faith to prayer.

For being a friend

My motive is not a reflex
Reaction looking for sex
That is the least of all
Reason for me to fall
In love with somebody
Also, that would be shoddy
Yet I am not as pure
As somebody's tear
Tho what I have saved
Doubtless does help love to pave
Through the part a little gaudy
Of somebody
When to come to where I am going
Somebody's love will be flowing
Then I shall slow down
For likely I am to drown
Yet I hear the sound
Of somebody found
Touched to the quick
Somebody shall stick
With me everywhere
Will we go there
Where there is not fear
There is where I shall see not tear
Nor more sin
For being a friend
A position so knobbly
When you love somebody.

LETTERS TO LEIGH

A little sorrow

I cannot forget your taste
The taste that I still do not waste
You are sweet like sugar
lips that do fit as my cigar
Then sneaking kisses out of doors
Only made me ready for more
Kissing in the elevator
Then made me feel better
In between each passing floor
Was too hard to ignore
For if we had been caught
We had then trouble bought
If them we so fought
More then we had sought
things are different now
Yet I taste you somehow
Upon my tongue
Then I grow numb
To any other thing
For your thought does bring
A little sorrow
With the taste that I borrowed
Yet I do not allow sweet to grow bitter
Because I would think that it be fitter
To come to you now
Find you somehow
Come to you alone
Then embrace you until home.

LETTERS TO LEIGH

I hope for you to take me into your heart

I have to stay away from my pen
For I am finding that I send
My one thought
With all of its fault
Toward your direction
For your inspection
Of any defect
For me to then reflect
Upon
As I am so doing there is one
Thought
That I hope to send
For my heart I hope you to mend
Before that thought does depart
I hope for you to take me into your heart
For you and I in love are one another's twin
Only together may we win
If ever we separate our heart
Lost will be a part
Yet if I use my head
To help love instead
In keeping our heart whole
Also our soul
Mine is the double
Of your own, soap bubble
Yet I am not to blame
For having gifted you that name
For soon our love shall have fame.

LETTERS TO LEIGH

If I am right or wrong

Do I ever hesitate
To take my pen then state
That tis true love for you that I feel
Yes, for you my heart does kneel
Your love from him I would steal
That then my heart may heal
If I am right or wrong
Will fight I hard and long
To again hear you sing that song
Even if in the pressing throng
Yes, life may again be fair
When I am in your stare
I am yet still in the race
To say this to your face
Is it not enough that I should love
Now I have found that I must prove
That you are still my little dove
Above my heart you do rove
With that you may fillet
Then say
Place upon a tray
Is it yours for the taking
Yes, it is there for the shaking
Yet, if there is not love to be making
Only do not take it for breaking
If you do not know what you have been missing
Just take it solely for kissing.

LETTERS TO LEIGH

Yet we are all alone

Your memory is still distinct
My love for you is not extinct
Once you said that I was bone of your bone
In that thought you are not alone
In thinking that way
Because I do tell you today
That I so feel the same
Except my heart does feel lame
Yet you may heal
If only should you feel
That it is proper and necessary
To use loves apothecary
I will take what you prescribe
Then listen to your diatribe
For I shall be the best patient
If love for him you leave vacant
Also use loves healing herb
By your choice of each word
I will make a fast recovery
Then you will make a discovery
That through it all
My love shall
Be waiting on my nurse
To remove this lonely curse
I do not have you yet
Tho one day I will hold and pet
We are bone of our bone
Yet we are all alone.

LETTERS TO LEIGH

Happily I was blind

In the valley of my love
does sit a quite cove
Protected on each lone side
From loves changing tide
The mountains all around
Do mellow out the echo of loves sound
There I am left mute
Before loves gentle flute
On top was loves fountain
Then scaled I loves mountain
This time the first
To cure my thirst
There I stayed for awhile
Without any guile
Filling my belly
With loves sweet jelly
There I stayed for several days
Then found myself in loves maze
My way out I could not find
Happily I was blind
Yet I found the maze unfinished
Tho my love was not diminished
Then I came back down to my nook
For other love I did not look
Came I back down to my valley
I did not stroll, I could not salley
Down I came with head held low
For my heart another blow.

LETTERS TO LEIGH

Forever there would be my love

The cloud today
That brought to you rain
Does not delay
To bring for me pain
I am glad you are brought cool relief
Yet I am bothered beyond belief
To shower love on you as you cried
I would ride
Upon the healing winds
Then I would send love to you to mend
Your wounded spirit
I should do this so that you may feel it
Then keep love flowing with that falling sound
Until love closed every heartfelt wound
I then would treat any silent scar
From afar
That your heart
Would be one part
When I was done
Your soul would be won
Then ready
For my wind that is steady
Then for my rain
To lessen the pain
Forever there would be my love
Sent from above
To all of this I would soon softly add bliss
If I rode upon the wind and a cloud, that is.

LETTERS TO LEIGH

I think that you will find

If you do not know that I love you by now
I shall just have to love you more somehow
I find myself thinking more yet I just draw a blank
Truly I love you and into love I have sank
Up over my head
Not to my neck instead
If there were any way possible
Then my love would be more lovable
Yet you may see that it is endurable
I happily think, if only you were more havable
As I am writing my heart out
For you I still pout
This is about all that I am able to do
The only way that I have to woo
I could run an add in your paper
To see if there may be an answer
For this love that has shown
With true love for you it is known
I should only have to wait until you turned the
page
When you saw it your love would take the stage
Then say to you, return
Toward whom you once gently spurned,
There in your love I would churn
Until your love for me you learned
I am almost at the end of this book
Like my heart, it is open to inside look
I think that you will find
I do love you with heart, soul, and mind.

LETTERS TO LEIGH

Thou holy spirit is everywhere

My father who art in heaven
Only thou do know what I am feeling
Thou knowest if my heart does need healing
Thou knowest if her love I am stealing
I am ready to lay down my wand
Then leave all in thine hand
Thou made all time and thereof the sand
Particles without number in the land
I try to write this without pride
For in thy shadow I hope to hide
With thou belongeth all decision
Which sometime cut like an incision
I am thy son and thou knowest best
To keep me from temptation lest
I should somewhere fall
Where I would fail to heed thy angels call
Thou comfortest me with thy staff and rod
Then bringest me what thou wilt with thy nod
Thou art my father above creation
It is thou who chastiseth nations
Who am I that thou seeest my situation
Who am I that thou art my salvation
To thou alone I offer prayer
That thy angels bring up the stairs
Thou holy spirit is everywhere
Tho we only see through air
Blessed be thou and thy holy son
For he in turn blesses everyone.

LETTERS TO LEIGH

Results of temptation

I would write more in regard to him
But I know that he does see through my sham
Of that I am not ashamed
For he does know that I am not to blame
Because sin entered man through a liar
Then is in us through Adam our sire
Yet the judgement receiver
Is Satan the deceiver
He was a liar from the start
Then from heaven did depart
He wanted to become God of this world
Yet the Lords flag still flies unfurled
At his feet all lay curled
Until in the pit Satan is hurled
Then we will know joy untold
While the final chapter unfolds
We will know then why it had to be God's son
To come down from heaven then die for everyone
For that is the route
That with him did sprout
From a world of sighs
Back to paradise
I cannot say it all
Only on him may call
He will not deny me
Yet he will let me see
Without hesitation
The results of temptation.

LETTERS TO LEIGH

I can never pay thou back enough

Lord tho I have started on a higher climb
I cannot just leave Leigh behind
She was with me through thick and thin
And we repent if twas sin
Yet thou knowest her heart she did lend
 I am glad to call her friend
May she be a friend of thine
 please help her to walk the line
Please watch over us at night
For we are precious in thy sight
Although I love her
For thou I reserve my highest honour
I can never pay thou back enough
Or thank thou for thy gentle cuff
As I was saying before
My love for Leigh is hard to ignore
Yet next to thou hers is nothing
For both of us thou art soothing
Of all my sins I do repent
Regarding her please relent
Please on her let my love be spent
Down to every last feeling sent
That for thou I do not reserve
Whose love I do not deserve
Yet if I have found favour in thine eyes
Then if I have been noticed avoiding lies
Thou may give us to each other
For thou a little thing and not much bother.

Will my heart stay low

Leigh
I love thee
Tis plain to see
That you love me
I just cannot forget
That love will yet
Let us come
Together as one
You need not remind
That your love I shall find
Yes I will wait
At your gate
For you to come out
After your pout
Is changed from a frown
Into upside down
A smile you may call
It if you call it at all
Tho to me it
Is my heart bit
When
You grin
I do not know
I may be slow
Yet my love does flow
I want it to show
Will my heart stay low
Only you may know.

A love for a friend

Against all advice
Some call it a vice
Like throwing the dice
Yet I call them mice
Then with my hard head
I do the opposite instead
This pen I keep shoving
My love I keep loving
As I hold open the door
For those that I ignore
Who do not understand
A love for a friend
My old friends altogether
May stand out in the weather
I shall take my place
Next to your face
I want none other
Not sister nor brother
Your love is not the same
Although they are not to blame
It is without hesitation
That you give me resuscitation
This love is silent
Tho a torment
To hold alone
While I wait on the phone
As the soothsayer sayeth
I must have faith.

LETTERS TO LEIGH

My only hope

My heart will feel pert
When you stop the hurt
It shall then feel better
Tho now it is wetter
Because of my tears
Which cover it my dear
When may I bring you on home
Where I now sit all alone
Why do you never call
Making my face to fall
My only hope
Is to cope
With the knowledge
That your love I may pillage
For when that day does come
You shall not run
Toward the wrong direction
Is my prediction
You will not be late
As you run straight
Into my hands
I do hope and plan
To love you dear
Without the fear
That you will leave
Me to grieve
I know that you are coming
One day into my arms running.

LETTERS TO LEIGH

Of what is fine

I am your spirit warrior
Working and fighting for your
Love to stay in my life
By combating strife
That does come by every day
To snare you in any way
Evil ever does dare
For it is in the air
How I treat another
Helps any who would be my spiritual brother
Overcome those
Who would battles for good lose
I am fighting for any friend
Also all good men
By treating
Badness in any human
As influenced by a demon
If I give into bad
I shall know then that I had
Lost a chance
For the defence
Of what is fine
For example if I am lying
I myself injure
Although being good does conjure
Our demons to go away
Back to hell where they shall stay.

LETTERS TO LEIGH

Only one may stop loves flow

You are gone
Yet my love does live on
Yes it is still growing
Constant love is showing
What it has always shown
That in love with you I am known
 your love has not flown
 nor is our love blown
It is just going to take some time
For you to feel that you are mine
I do not know about the do or the do not
I only know about my want
I prefer to say my need
That I feel as my heart does bleed
Only one may stop loves flow
For this is how my hearts love must show
It may withstand any blow
For it one day may know
That you will be back
Then of love there shall be none to lack
Until then
I do not feel that it be a sin
For me to keep writing
To keep loves lamp lighting
Does it matter who is right
As long as I hold you into the night
Right or wrong
I long to hear your song.

LETTERS TO LEIGH

How my love to you must fly

It does make me feel better
To write to you each letter
Please try not me to blame
If they light an old flame
I know that you may feel the same
When me your mind does name
I am not doing much
Just staying in touch
With your feeling
That emotional healing
Which on my heart is sealing
While life is dealing
All and every card
That make it so hard
To do without
My love fount
Do you see now
As time does pass by
How my love to you must fly
I know that my card
Is not far
From the middle
Of loves riddle
If I am not to beat
Could I not cheat
To improve my chance
that your love does enhance.

LETTERS TO LEIGH

Should you take what I could bring

I was looking at some earrings
Only some triflings
They matched your eyes
Yes, they were just your size
It was with regret
That I them let
Stay where they were
For they were not a cure
Because I was sure
That they would not get me anywhere
All for you I would buy
Only to feel your sigh
I should present to you a diamond ring
If I could only hear you sing
I would give you anything
Should you take what I could bring
The impulse was hard to ignore
As I was headed toward the door
Yet for you I did want more
That I may do, I am sure
Then I went to another store
There for it I was too poor
I shall come back another day
To put my love on lay-a-way
I care not what you say
Your price I am willing to pay
If it will bring a ray
Near your heart to stay.

LETTERS TO LEIGH

All may watch and stare

 The voices drew near unto my ear one day, I
thought with demonic play
Tho they could not here long delay for the Lord
sent then on their way
 yet what now my tame thoughts say
Do change from day to day
For one thing does the same stay
 they wish for you to be in my word-play
The only voice that is within myself does tell me to
be kind
How others often do not to bring to mind
If you should feel it
You may call it Holy Spirit
Tis around for all to feel
When you offer yourself for it in to dwell
It will help during a bad spell
Leading you back through hell
It does amaze all and every doctor
Because it does good mental health foster
Some make as their aim
For their illness to blame
That is all good and fine
Only keep looking for the sign
That the spirit does dwell in you
For it may kindly help when feeling blue
All may watch and stare
I know that the spirit is in the air
When you are in need of some healing
Just search out that special feeling
That all men hope to find
To ease the anguish of the mind

LETTERS TO LEIGH

I do not know where everyone else mind has dwelt
As for myself, within and without, I have the Holy
Spirit felt.

LETTERS TO LEIGH

It was then to my relief

Did you want me to cry
Baby I did try
That drop may know that I yet shall bring you
home
My tear I did not shed
Because my love you have led
My soul have you fed
Maybe to have left yours poor instead
For the sake of your own my tear did not come
Now my heart has bled
Love purest red
I love you, I have said
Do not please call our love dead
I have led you around the lawn
To have kept our love from fallen
My tear kept on stalling
Even when you were bawling
Your tears were such
That my heart they did touch
 it was then to my relief
That your tears were brief
Now I feel my own moving around
Then my ears may hear the sound
Of my own weeping coming on
A tear for myself I disown
Because I have forgotten the liquid blue
Yet the colour of my eyes I now wash out for you
Yet if that was done
I would realize then that I was only one.

LETTERS TO LEIGH

Down deep inside

Were you surprised
When I lied
To him about loving you
You do know that it was not true
That lie I have began to rue
Because now I have not anyone to
Blame
That lie is my own shame
I only wrote that letter
To make it easy and better
For you to live together
Yet now my eyes are wetter
Because you do know that I want you for my own
In your wedding gown
Until death do us part
To shop at the love mart
Deep down inside
I do know that you will be my bride
I need you to be my wife
For the rest of my life
I shall give you all that you want
If my dreams you will haunt
If that letter
Has your heart inside of a fetter
I take it all back
My love you do not lack
I shall see you one day
For there will be my heart to pay.

LETTERS TO LEIGH

That would be a small price to pay

You are not a material girl
Yet you do like for your hair to curl
You like material things
With the pleasure that they bring
I am not rich yet
Still, I am willing to make a bet
That I shall be ready to buy
For you that what makes you sigh
You are not a material girl
Yes, you are only my plain old Earle
Tho it is a material world
At that my money I shall hurl
To make you happy in some way
That would be a small price to pay
I do know that some day
You may pay me back and lay
Your love down
Without a frown
As I take you to town
To buy you a gown
You are not material I know
For you let your love show
Even if I have no
Money to blow
Because until the end
Your love did send
To me your friend
Your love did lend.

LETTERS TO LEIGH

Underneath loves fount

I will not have it said
That our love is dead
Although we are apart
Loves dart
By chances art
Still does make me one part
One half
Of a love bath
Do not even say
Nor ever play
In that way
For there is coming a day
When love shall pay
Then we will be allowed to play
Our hearts out
Underneath loves fount
Until we are all clean
Then we will know what love does mean
We shall stand arm-in-arm
Safe from all harm
As we feel love move in the air
Between our stare
As we gaze
Love will start to blaze
To fan the flame
Shall we be to blame
For falling into the fire
Is loves desire.

LETTERS TO LEIGH

Whatever you do, wherever you are

I am going to roll my love up inside of this paper
For in my heart thy love does still caper
You will never be alone
Because love does make our two hearts one
Whatever you do, wherever you are
You shall know that you are loved from afar
Not just once, not just twice
You are always precious in my eyes
As you rise up out of the bed
Try to keep this inside of your head
That for you my heart has bled
Oh please let it be said
That while we were apart
I did keep a loving heart
What it does say is true
For I am in love with you
As you do each daily chore
Keep your eyes up off of the floor
Keep on looking up above
For with you there is one in love
Who does want to be with you all through the day
To help you please in any way
I do not have much more to say
Yet I just cannot wait until the day
When I see upon you a grin
Then a smile all over again
It shall not be a sin
If we let love win.

LETTERS TO LEIGH

I am dying a death that is soft

Now it is June the first
For your love I still thirst
I do not want any run-a-round
Only I need your love safe and sound
I know that you have a good song
You know that I do not do anything wrong
Like the flame and the moth
I am dying a death that is soft
If my heart does fly near
Winged love you may sear
That I could endure
If only you called me dear
Are you not a towering fire
The object of my desire
If you do call me a liar
I shall prepare to fly higher
To up above the smoke
 for a better look
Then dive right into
That blazing inferno
Do I not need to escape
Yet want I only just a taste
Of the love that I am missing
Which is still hissing
You may take my every wing
If for me you shall sing
In the flame I will be
With fire soft all around me.

LETTERS TO LEIGH

I am living not a fable

Our love is on the table
My wits are almost stable
However others do label
I am living not a fable
Like the blind mice
You shall not have to ask me twice
We are supposed to be one another's friend
Yet my heart you do rend
Because you do not lend
Your love on me to mend
My heart that is broken
Which has become a token
That is being well spent
By and for love to you sent
Your love for me I do feel
For my heart has come close to heal
Whatever life does deal
Take my heart and peel
Like a cantaloupe
That I may learn to cope
For your love I will forever scope
Surely your heart I may one day rope
Then tie in so many a knot
That our past
Will the more fast
Be forgot
We shall then begin a tour
Of our loves future.

LETTERS TO LEIGH

In my need

Is it only a matter of time
Before again that you are mine
This thought I do find
Is good for my mind
It will, I know, come true
If I keep on loving you
If unable I am to continue
The tears shed will not be a few
Yet if I am to make a selection
I hope to avoid depression
Whether I will stand or fall
Shall depend on whether you love me at all
May unworthy thoughts cease
I say over and over then please
I know that you cannot see
Me
In my need
Yet you are the seed
From which love does grow
Maybe you should know
What I am to say
What am I to do
To how do I love pay
Then how do I you woo
As you have been a while away
For a while I have had to stay
Will you come back
To join me in a love attack.

LETTERS TO LEIGH

My love did bloom

Am I yet under some influence
Of your slight nuance
When I do talk
As everywhere that I walk
Your flavour
I do still savour
Your conversation
Still is enchanting
Your love wizard
Once had a lonely visage
Yet that you changed
For that first time you sang
My love did bloom
Then my soul made room
For you it to join
 two sides of a coin
We became
May as such therein we place our name
Are we now apart
Yet love will start
For it has came that to fix
For you shall be a nix
I am so fully confident
That your smile so radiant
Will become ever near
For mine to mirror
Then between that space
We shall make for love a face.

LETTERS TO LEIGH

Am I not down on my knee

Are we all addicted to something
Am I addicted to your loving
Will I not take no for an answer
Shall I yet listen to any fancier
Way of ending
The love that I am sending
For you to have at your leisure
With pleasure
From you toward me a glance
Does become to my heart a lance
From your lips a word
Comes into my inner part as a sword
Yet I will behave
If love you shall save
It is so easy to ask how
Only just pierce it now
I do aim to plead
Am I not down on my knee
Is there any way
For me to save the day
Give a one and only hint
I shall be forever bent
On carrying that thought thru
Just only for you
I know that I may be able to do so
If loves light should yet glow
Within your heart
While we are apart.

LETTERS TO LEIGH

Could it be that you are the woman of my life

As long as the words yet come
Our love is not done
I love you a lot
Not only in one spot
Your face is from an artist easel
From nimble lip to eye of hazel
To keep you from that frown
Let us not forget your hair light brown
Which does fall like lace
About that pixie face
  that ever looks quite snappy
Also, you always make me happy
Could it be that you are the woman of my life
I hope that we shall be man and wife
If I could then I would write better
To hear you say that I need not, should make my
eyes less wetter
One day in time your love I shall own
When you do wear our wedding gown
I will think that it is also part mine
For then will be a special time
As you approach from the aisle
We shall both have on that benevolent smile
Then as we say we do,
We shall continue to woo
Because we have each paid all that was due
As debtors to love we did not lose
After we have pledged that wedding vow
Love will be forever stronger, somehow.

LETTERS TO LEIGH

For when you love somebody

As this pen I must shove
All of these thoughts of love
Keep bubbling upward and forth
Toward you for all that they are worth
One then all each seem to say
That my heart at your feet does lay
Also, they do seem to say,
Always my love is the same every day,
For to you I do pay
My love in such a lonely way
With all of this much similar thought
I find that I have weakly fought
Nor have I searched or sought
Any thought of another ought
 for I am without a reason to fight
These thoughts that are so full of light
For when you love somebody
You will not think a thought that is shoddy
To your love I have opened each eye
My love that I feel for you that I will not deny
Take my eyes along with my soul
For without you I am not yet whole
I shall settle for not anything less
Than to be with you and your bliss
For your love I find that I am in a battle
Say that you love me, I will not tattle
Do not leave me after you have planted in my
heart loves seed
Especially when it has just only began to bleed.

LETTERS TO LEIGH

I do love my love fount

It is eight o'clock
Your love lays in a lock
Around your heart is the cruel stock
That is as hard as a rock
I must find the key
For the one who I call me
I will leave not a stone
That I shall not overturn
Not ever even one
Perhaps, to my ruin
I have not been known
For my love to be shown
Yet without a hint of a doubt
I do love my love fount
What may I do
While I cannot woo
You
Besides to be a fool
As I am holding this tool
Should I be supposed to remain cool
For lack of a fitting thought, I am not
Yes, I am in a way hot
Thus a little mad
Added to that, I am sad
Somewhat blue
Over you
While crying a little
Over loves riddle.

LETTERS TO LEIGH

Yet one heart

Our love is not extinct
Tho it does come near that brink
We did save it with a smile
While know we that love has its own wile
We may still somehow yet figure
That we are in a way together
Although still apart
Yet one heart
Still not quite whole
Likened to our soul
For like our heart
We in the past took a part
 that we then well hid
Until we may say that we have rid
Our hearts of desire
For false fire
As we hang our head lowly
The more to watch time pass by slowly
We yet know that one day
 we may be able to say
All of what was lost
Has been sought for and bought by the cost
The price that we have paid
Was our love so down laid
Yet love did churn
Thus floating from thence to return
To us as one another's lover
Yet sister and brother.

LETTERS TO LEIGH

You are still my hope so fond

I did not write to you yesterday
I did have the time to play
Yet I could not find very much to say
Forgive me, for I left it that way
Now I find that I have to do more
Than I did even before
If ever my soul was sore
I must forever dig down to the core
Down to the forgotten lore
There I shall find good words galore
To touch your soul then test the bottom
That you have almost forgotten
If only I may make this love stand
I would take you unto dreamland
Into the land of your origin
Where every dream does come from
I could await you there with my secret name
Where I would make my intent your heart to tame
As we watched a mythological creature
Steadily I should compare your every feature
As I watch for your frown
While you would gaze around
If that I ever should see
I would then bring you back to reality
Toward my love would be my hope
If that was so, then with my reality I could cope
You are still my hope so fond
Here I put my hope into my wand.

LETTERS TO LEIGH

I shall someday be holding you

As ever, this has been a long day
While looking for a word that may pay
Sometimes it does seem to happen that way
Even when I do have something to say
My name may include the third
Yet still I cannot find the word
To melt the ice that does surround your heart
For a fire into there to start
Then inside that place
Beneath your lace
I have made entry into this race
At a steady pace
If every day on my scroll I average two
I shall someday be holding you
If only you may read this
I know not whether you would either shed tears or
find bliss
Perhaps the two should go hand in hand
Until times glass of sand
Does finish every particle
For by then we may have signed that marriage
article
I know that God is not cruel
To myself, I seem not to feel like a fool
Neither do I feel blue
When I think of loving you
Even if all were some jest
I have tasted love of the best
Yet I am to be careful lest
God should end my love fest.

LETTERS TO LEIGH

I should not find love a chore

If you were water then you might be my pond
To dip there into your love I would be so fond
For once I would lay down my wand
Then I could wade softly amidst each delicate
frond
I would not want that your love should be tangled
Nor for your emotions to be tangled
Should I not take care to misuse?
Or emotionally abuse
For this delicate environment
Must be with me into our retirement
My soul should find refreshment
Just standing on your embankment
Where if my heart was to bleed
Or perhaps if I felt the need
I could merely touch your weed
That would then become hopes seed
You should naturally have a waterfall
With waters gurgling call
If I should come close I shall
Hear the sirens in their hall
Melt my heart they would
If melt more it could
That would ease once they had learned
Loves love already my heart churned
Away from you I could not be tore
With me you would never bore
I should not find love a chore
Then my heart could not be sore.

LETTERS TO LEIGH

All love without pride

Playing like a child
May my words meek and mild
Open closed doors
Of from where love pours
Open one then take a peek
To see if it is the one that I seek
Then come outside to play
I shall try again another day
Love will not delay
Shall not love find a way
Then hang about in loves yard
There to run around until I am tired
Finally, I come back to loves house
Just as quiet as a mouse
Then I attempt to wake love up
To drink from that sweet loves cup
Yet love is still asleep
I try not to weep
Then not to be idly slow
Me, myself, and I do try the window
Always careful not to fall
I am only looking for love that is all
Then I have to leave again
Yet on that place about my face just a trace of a
big grin
As long as it is not a sin
Love will still win
Again I am outside
All love without pride.

LETTERS TO LEIGH

I will take my time

Have love, may travel
If your love I do unravel
I am in anticipation
To timely arrive at my destination
I will not tire
For I have the wheels of desire
I shall drive slow
For I do not want my tire to blow
Yet if I do drive fast
I could say that I am here at last
I will take my time so as to enjoy the ride
Coming back you shall be by my side
I have found that if I use every gear
I am always able to shift my fear
That am you I losing
While I am cruising
Then I shall hurry every chance that I get
For I know that you know me and yet
I will take my time
While enjoying your scenery so fine
Thus I shall hurry along
For I miss the sound of your song
I will keep driving on straight ahead
For I know that our love is not dead
If I shall be stopped along the way
I will know just what I am to say
When I finally do reach you wherever you are
I shall say join me for love will take us far.

LETTERS TO LEIGH

To hold near

I have about two-hundred page
All of my love wage
Pledged from my hearts stage
Yet still my love does rage
Within my heart
Where it did start
From the beginning
Then keeps on sending
These thoughts of love
For your glove
To pick up
Into your cup
 to hold near
While having not fear
Of breaking
This love that we are making
Together
Despite the weather
Which is hot
That is not
What I wanted
As my love vaunted
Into your lap
To tap
The sap
Then map
Out the way
 toward loves best day.

LETTERS TO LEIGH

Yet I never know

I have poetry in my every dream
Love is in my lonely vein
Let me this paper stain
Ere I become insane
In my dream
I rehearse
Of love a deep scene
Or loves curse
When I awaken
I find that I am taking
Any line
That is fine
Then shake I this pen
With my heart open
To put on paper
Words that caper
All about
They then come out
With a mute shout
Through my love fount
When I am done
I know that I have won
Another bout
With my dreams pout
Yet I never know
If you will show
That you give ear
 hearken to my stumbling tear.

LETTERS TO LEIGH

My torment

This feeling may come from loving your look
More than my every book
Which I have forsook
Since my heart you took
Alone it would not have left
Even for your cleft
Yet it was your total
That made me into a model
Loving man
Of you a fan
If I may win a prize
I would wish that it could be your eyes
Upon
One
As lonely
 such as me
Since you left
Me bereft
Of every sense
Only your taste still does rinse
Around my tongue
Which yet soaks it as a sponge
I wish that my any word
Would fly like a bird
Into your ear
For so then you could hear
My torment
 that haunts each moment.

Love is what I am talking about

Now I am pacing
Soon I will be racing
On my way to tracing
Your heart for unlacing
I must start
On the hardest part
Of your heart
To there apply loves dart
Love is what I am talking about
For that I shall take any route
To take me there
Where
your love does begin
For tis not a sin
For me you to love
To give love a gentle shove
Into the right direction
Before the day of inspection
When we will see
If our hearts still do bleed
For one another
Over each other
For love we must have hope
How others cope
I do not know
For that I cannot do
Yet as for the future of us
We shall not cuss.

LETTERS TO LEIGH

I am showing you all of my feeling

I make love to you when I rise at dawn
After making love to you while I am lying down
In the time between
My heart does toward you lean
As I go about loves chore
I think of you who does not bore
Before the day is done
I know that your love is newly won
I do not watch television much
For I am looking too much for your touch
Around here there is a lot of noise
From a total of five little boys
With all of their toys
Yet all that I am hearing is your voice
As I write these words I do sit
Feeling that soon I shall stand to miss you a little
bit
I would rather have had you then fall
Than never to come to know love at all
I am showing you all of my feeling
That you have on my heart been sealing
I love you as I do my own soul
Which one day you then may know
That it is not nearly whole
For that am I a fool
I do not think so
Surely these words of love shall do
If with them I cannot hope
How shall I forever cope.

LETTERS TO LEIGH

My heart as of yet does remain tore

My true medicine
Is you my friend
To
Do
Without
Does make my mind pout
My feeling
Of this heart swelling
Ever does find me then sends me to hell
When you are away for a spell
Now that you have been gone
For so long
Is it wrong
To not hear your song
As it used to be so free
Like the sound of a bird
With that of a bee
Yet it I have not heard
In a century
Certainly
You may spare
Some love fare
For a lone ear
Touch but one eye
So that I may bear
My constant sigh
While if my love this may bore
My heart as of now does yet remain tore.

LETTERS TO LEIGH

To forever, as time has the sand

I keep sensing deja-vu
My every thought does again find you
It is not to matter how much that they do
They only do make me more willing to woo
These thoughts of you are often frantic
More often that sometime my reflections of you do
put me into a panic
I cannot find words enough
That would melt a heart as yours so tough
Yet it does what it has to
Like I have to keep loving so true
You may say that I am in retreat
Yet I shall never admit defeat
For as long that I find a pen within my hand
To forever, as time has the sand
If still there are ocean and land
You may be my woman
Even if you continue to frown
Twill be a smile once each other we do own
Our love once then for all
When we heed loves call
Then you may unclose each ear
For I will soothe then calm your fear
All and any of them love will allay
On that beautiful day
For this I am faithful to pray
With hope that love will stay
For with us may love play
As we await smiles and of love a ray.

LETTERS TO LEIGH

When there are more than one sweet rose

Every rose
Does have a thorn
That we must know
For with one they are born
If to seek her you should dare
Handle with care
For you may be forlorn
If you touch one that is shorn
Thus you must risk a little hell
Then if into there you should fall
Allow her name to gently call
To lead you out the way
To find her sweet bouquet
Another problem does pose
When there are more than one sweet rose
How should you know which to choose
When to touch one that is right for you
Observe, please a bird with a bee
Do then they not kneel on a bended knee
Watch how they all do act
Then know and understand tact
When they have all flown away
Come on near
To stay
To take her by her thorn
Then yourself prepare
For so her seed of love at your touch will be born.

Because my love is deep

Happiness knows not any bound
Since my joy in you I have found
I will not wait another day
Nor shall I delay
To make a point
To keep us joint
At the heart
While we are apart
As a matter of fact
I need not tact
For all that I have to
Do
Is have you
To woo
Wherever you are
You will know that I care
Because my love is deep
I shall not always weep
There is a day to dawn
When your love will be shown
That I am in expectation
Of your salvation
While you I deliver
With able aid from cupids quiver
I cannot wait on the day
When I may say
That I love you
I am to you true.

LETTERS TO LEIGH

I have said it many times

Writing a poem is like going for a walk
I never know where to end my talk
Or where to turn around
As I listen for your sound
Because as with you I walk beside
I try to turn the tide
Toward my direction
Then upon inspection
I find that loves origin
Is with your vocal organ
Which I do love to hear
That I embrace so dear
As if I held you near
We would not know fear
I do know not where us this poem is taking
Yet along the way love is making
Us feel for each other
A love for one another
I have said it many times
Keep looking for loves sign
For that will lead you onto
path of a heart is for you.

LETTERS TO LEIGH

A new love flow

Yes there is a girl that I do love very much
Yet right now she is out of touch
For my good love she would vouch
Because my love is a love of such
Emotion
That she had the notion
For us to one day marry
Yet she does tarry
I am not known to terrorize
I just need to socialize
If you could you may admit
That you have an old love that you cannot quit
Yet we could get together
Then come hell then bad weather
We would have someone
To call our own
What we have in the past
May still last and last
Inside of our heart
Where love did start
For if they come back one day
To them we may go play
Tho if they do not
We should each give a shot
Toward getting to know
A new love flow
We need not forget
Love that our hearts have felt.

LETTERS TO LEIGH

Now I have my heart open

Of your love I shall take a slice
Go ahead then, give me twice
Of the amount that you would
Give if you could
Love me until
I ask for a refill
Then as love does pour
I will softly ask for more
While you are never done
You shall be forever won
Over toward my way
Leaning forward as I say,
Here I now stand empty
Asking you so simply
To empty your pot
As to give me a lot
Now I have my heart open
All of it is hoping
That your love shall return
For my love you will not spurn
That my heart shall not burn
For my love will ever churn
Inside deep down
Where true love is to be found
There we shall be bound
To sing loves sound
Only do not forget
To allow love to pour yet.

LETTERS TO LEIGH

When I ever think of you

I miss thee, I miss thou
I still do love you anyhow
Perhaps I am a fool
If not, maybe loves tool
I do not feel that I have been used
Yet I am kind of blue
When I ever think of you
Of our love so true
Tho I just cannot accept
Our love as a reject
It is too good
Is it not what it should
If possible more it would
Love more if it could
I am only one lonely half
Of our love bath
Please do not bid au-revoir
To that love reservoir
For unto my love fountain
My love does keep mounting
Let there be love yet
Not for nothing in loves net
For the world was made
To love in the shade
When then in the heat
To retreat
For to find shelter
There where love we pilfer.

LETTERS TO LEIGH

Another day

My love is not a smouldering ruin
For it may light me up soon
Love is not a disaster
For it is more like a flight of stairs
The more that are past
Only does mean that the longer love will last
Love is like grass growing
Tho to us the growth is not showing
For love is like a faithful pet
That will for you wait yet
Another day
While time does delay
For you I do pray
I say
Then begin
To sin
Again
My friend
Is it true that I am my own enemy
For I have laid my heart open only to be taken by
a den of thieves
Yet to you I will be faithful
While avoiding thoughts that are hateful
Just a fair thought and a glad emotion
Yet always to look for loves lotion
For that is good medicine
To cure the damage within
My life, my soul, my heart
Ending strife, making whole, and one part.

LETTERS TO LEIGH

I never meant for you any harm

My dull mind
Cannot find
The good word
That your love does deserve
About that I have thought
While I constantly sought
Then caught
Yet fought
Words for your inspection
Only for your direction
As I hold them near
Like I held you dear
I have not fear
That love will sear
Upon me a soft scar
For near and far
May it be known
Let it be shown
That I love you
So,
So
True
For to whom it may concern
I never meant for you any harm
Yet always I aid love and abet
If only these words I do let
Find their forgotten way
That they may say that love was made to stay.

LETTERS TO LEIGH

I began with only half of a chance

You shall always have a special place
Inside of my heart a tender space
From where I will trace
That very special face
Then decorate that with lace
For it would my heart brace
As I am in the world
Where if only you were in my arms curled
You do not need a special reason
Nor any noble season
I only want you to therein rest
While I pass all of your test
I just need to say as my last behest
Beware of my love fest
For if it does find you one day
You shall surely have love to pay
Love that is fine
Flowing with rhyme
Yet still looking for the sign
That love will one day be mine
I cannot express how much
That I do miss your gentle touch
Ask me if I do love you enough
Even when you are being tough
I began with only half of a chance
Just barely did we have one dance
Yet as we pass through the years
I shall never have my fill of tears.

LETTERS TO LEIGH

An emotional healing

I have two pages still
Two for you to fill
To you I try to sell
Two with words that tell
Your love is at my touch
There it is such
A feeling
An emotional healing
That I may give
While we live
You need not to grieve
Just in me believe
That today's flame
Will be the same
Tomorrow
Without sorrow
To borrow
Only to follow
Me, your man
Into a wonderland
Where shall we be glad
That we always had
Each other,
One another
To get through
Feeling blue
So
We will stay true.

Something to measure others upon

There is still a smile upon my face
Yet in my eye a trace
Of a tear
Only without the fear
Of turning blue
From losing you
You I cannot forget
For me you will not let
A day go past
Unless it is cast
Into my memory
That your love was free
From then to now it has become
Something to measure others upon
My love to you I dedicate
For that love for you does not hesitate
To let you know so fast
That our love is going to last
Within our heart
Where it did start
Then onto these pages
Written in stages
Finally unto my soul
Which became whole
After you became known
For then to me your love was shown
In that special way
What more am I able to say.

LETTERS TO LEIGH

The first stone has been cast

I have tried to make it all alone
Yet you are still bone of my bone
If you are without guilt then cast the first stone
Only do let my thoughts of love roam
 which was maybe I should find a new model
Then I could not find one poured from your mold,
all
That I thought was that I could make love
counterfeit
By writing of love that did not sit
In my heart
Still, I wanted a part
Of what I had lended
When writing of you I ended
Then I wrote of two ladies
Tho we were not steady
Because they did not appreciate
A poetic Johnny-come-too- late
I never wanted to stop writing of you
For I knew that our love was true
There I had reached an end
Of love words to send
Allow me to say that I only stopped then
As to make them the more precious to have been
Yet I do want to put it all in the past
Then write of love that will last
Be it slow or be it fast
The first stone has been cast
As long as my love does endure
I shall send to you a love that is pure.

LETTERS TO LEIGH

You may do to me not a greater wrong

It is my birthday
Did you remember today
Would it make any change
On the way that your heart does hinge
Let it open up
Then I may fill my cup
If so I shall drink my fill
Yet not, then I may be ill
I am not asking for much
Only a smile and a touch
Surely these you may spare
I think that would be fair
For you not to forget
That we may together be yet
Of all the nectar in the garden
I do want my flowers pardon
Even though I do stay up late
I still believe twill be my fate
To one day find you again
A lone way to find my friend
You may do to me not a greater wrong
Than to keep me from your song
If you do not know what I am trying to say
Allow me to say it another way
It has been some months and many a day
Yet my heart you do still slay
I would whisper into your ear
If only my love you wanted to hear.

LETTERS TO LEIGH

Back again into my arms

Come and pass a day
With me, for we shall play
As we used to
Do
Bring those days back
Sadness now I do not lack
Everywhere that I look
I am forsook
Now finding that I have not a sweet partner
To hold then share the heart of her
 all is void and what I now taste
Is the desolate waste
That my good love has come to
I do not even now want another to woo
They all may shoo, shoo, shoo
For all that I want is you
Back again into my arms
Safe from all alarm
Ever when you awaken
My love that has not forsaken
Shall cause you to lay still
As our heart does drink its fill
When the draughting is all done
Our love we may say has won
For you wished to pass a day
To bring for me a sunny ray
As it is not for to me to say
My love ever does say that you will stay.

LETTERS TO LEIGH

I wonder how many words there are left

Would you like to make a picture
Of my hearts fracture
How my blood does ever drop
How it may not ever stop
Of your love make for me a bandage
Because my heart does embrace loves bondage
Lay me down gently
Then say that you love me simply
For what I am
Please disregard my sham
From your feet upward may I look
To include into if I someday write a book
Therein may it be known
That my love toward you has flown
As people then turn any page
My love will show upon that stage
They will know that I am ill
Waiting on loves pill
Which only you may deliver
From the aid of cupids quiver
They shall all be suspended
To know how the story ended
Like myself
I wonder how many words there are left
Do I have worthy ammunition
For you to throw yourself upon
My love you may keep all of your armour
With due honour.

LETTERS TO LEIGH

For she has made it known

To know how to handle a woman
Learn how to hold her hand
As if dancing yet allow her to lead
Just hold hers like you are holding precious seed
When she does ever move in for a hug
Relax then your shoulders with a shrug
Forever still while holding her hand
Make not any demand
For your hug make sure
That your actions are pure
This will give her confidence
Enough to cross the fence
Into wanting to kiss
Which is hard to miss
Keep kissing her on the lip
Until she does want to sip
Then give her enough to drink
As she does reach the brink
 send your hands to feel
Her petulant nipple
Now is no time to rest
Fill your hands with breast
For she has made it known
That her blood is brought to foam
As you are hugging and kissing and feeling
With your senses reeling
 if you handle her right
You shall have a hot wax candle for the night.

LETTERS TO LEIGH

By love you are surrounded

Of love is there a wrong way
Do I have the right to stay
Down my heart I do lay
Nothing more may I say
Are there yet words that I have not found
That would please you with their sound
I would ask the birds to sing
My words with a pleasant ring
Has my heart not shed enough blood
Until it has become a flood
That you are in danger of drowning
While my heart is pounding
As the life preserver
Is also my love reservoir
Where you must take refuge
To escape loves deluge
Yet you are still not safe there
For that is where
My love does begin
To love again
By love you are surrounded
Because upon loves shore you are floundered
My love you cannot escape
For it must take every shape
To keep you reminded
That by love I am blinded
Yet my love shall seek you out
Even though your stronghold is stout.

LETTERS TO LEIGH

I am waiting on my woman

As I lie here on my bed
I find that enough has not been said
Of us two
Then I do feel blue
I would like to change
Yet all on you does hinge
My past, present, and future
Does depend upon another creature
Maybe life will drive
You to make me alive
You have shed tears before
Now just my love adore
I will spare you any tear
If you would only overcome that fear
Just come be my wife
The centre of my life
Of children, we shall have a few
While greeting each day anew
My soul may be your mirror
So to your own it may grow nearer
My life without you is like a connect the dots
With love missing in spots
Also it is like a jig-saw puzzle
That my mind cannot juggle
Yet out of the ashes the phoenix always must
arise
Behind her the nix is there to surprise
Do not ask me to a party join
I am waiting on my woman.

LETTERS TO LEIGH

Then out of all the confusion

I have not the grace
Nor the touch of lace
To unfasten your love
Then hold it in my glove
Yet with my clumsy style
I would lead you up the aisle
Then along with my touch
I would vouch
That for you I feel something beyond
Than what love is usually called upon
If that I could speak
Closely to your cheek
I would probably not need
To sow loves seed
If in this poor way
I may continue to say
Words that heal
That have loves appeal
I might soon win
Your heart again
Yet I always fall short
Then hope that you are a good sport
Enough to invite me back
To attempt again where I lack
For something that I cannot find
Then out of all the confusion
You are still my conclusion.

LETTERS TO LEIGH

Only for you I do concentrate

I have not jealousy
Only a bended knee
Am I not slow in every word
Yet mightier than the sword
I am not trying to blow your mind
For I have found that it is fine
You have never seen me at my best
Then I may be able to impress
You have seen my humble self
Also the few wits that I had left
When we were so alive
There by each others side
You made me into a different person
When apart I had a curse on
Myself alone cannot win
For in our soul we are one another's twin
These words cannot apply justice
To the hearts ice
That has covered up
A once love cup
Maybe I cannot say words like they are meant to
be
Baby, that is just me
I have never wished that I was him
His memory to me is dim
Only for you I do concentrate
Hoping you for me God will compensate
If I avoid any deadly sin
Including jealousy, which is one of them

LETTERS TO LEIGH

One day we shall drink a toast

I have so much to say
Yet I do not know the way
As I go I use caution
For I think of any notion
That may help to have proved
To you that you are the only woman that I ever
loved
Maybe now it has become known
Forever love for me you have shown
Yet you remembered
Then that you being so encumbered
We had to say ado
Tho I still love you
Where may I find
One of your kind
Another girl will not do
It is only you that I have to woo
Another would not claim me as their own
Nor have a special song
As my love may always run through this hearts
sieve
I still do yet believe
That in the course of time
Your hand will become mine
Shall I have you totally
That whole personality
That is what must remain important to me
What God has gave to you for free
One day we shall drink a toast
Then I will show that I love you most.

LETTERS TO LEIGH

If only my wife you were to be made

I feel the love that must move to shame
Any other loving flame
No love may come near
To what I do feel for you, dear
Others may try, others may fail
Yet I have found my holy grail
I have searched for you all of my life
Again I do choose you to be my wife
My cross I have had to bare
Now my load is as light as air
For since the Lord did touch me with his staff
I now go through life with a laugh
Waiting for your love to lay down
I forever wait for you without a frown
Of my flesh I have paid a pound
Yet you do not hear my complaining sound
For since your love I have found
Small has grown my hearts wound
I shall keep writing each letter
Until I find a way to make love better
As I begin I ask God please
Let all of my unworthy thoughts cease
He does answer me in his way
By giving me these words to say
He does call all of his sheep by name
For he loves us all the same
Yet my crown I would trade
If only my wife you were to be made.

LETTERS TO LEIGH

To find that nothing has changed

This is what may become of little boys who do not
sleep
They lay awake at night then allow their heart to
weep
Finally one may some day grow up to write a song
Of a love where he cannot belong
Yet from time to time there is a miracle
Of that I do need a particle
I may have the words that soothe and tear
Tho for them I need the lady to be near
That she may hear
Of this love that I rear
Up upon all alone
Waiting for her to climb there -on
As I say my prayers at night
I do pray for his guiding light
To watch over you over there
As my love is carried through the air
I do know that you make it day by day
Because that is what I hope when I pray
The Lord will rejoin us in his own good time
It is now up to me to hold the line
This I am so doing
With these letters that are wooing
You in advance
Of our meeting by chance
Which up above will be arranged
To find that nothing has changed
I still love you
As I used to do.

LETTERS TO LEIGH

I now raise my bid

Am I allowed to make up in some way
For still loving you today
There is something that I must confess
By your love I am yet possessed
Not just a small amount
Tis a great gushing love fount
Where I daily take a swim
There-in my wits grow dim
I find then you wading, making that smiling face
In that sunny place
There I am soaked through
With a love so smooth
That I am able to only think
To make myself shrink
For to let there be more
Of you to adore
Yet sooner or later I must come out
Tho I always leave on my love fount
Then I may have a little cry
Holding tears back, I then my eyes dry
Because I do love you so
For that feeling I cannot leave or let go
Though that is what I did
I now raise my bid
I would give all that I have
To feel your love salve
Would if I may with only these words take you by force
That one thought do I endorse.

LETTERS TO LEIGH

Because the love does flow on

The copy that I have of your smile
Is the original
Even a duplicate would show that you have not
guile
You are incorrigible
To my heart
Where my eyes start
To see you as you are
A cool burning fire
Then in the blink of an eye
I may think of a lie
Yet to you that I cannot tell
For I would save myself from that hell
When we were with each other
I was your lover and brother
Yet we had not incest
For we were far from that test
Then flying away to be free
Like two birds into a tree
Back to the ground to watch a cloud
Often talking loud
Then one day we saw a rainbow
Thought you that it was a special show
From there to the end
We stayed one another's friend
With only that one hitch
That both of our hearts needed a stitch
Because the love does flow on
Like blood drops onto a stone.

LETTERS TO LEIGH

Because love is to be found there

No one may feel my guilt, my shame
I am still drawn to you, old flame
 I cannot make myself get over
My friend and lover
Shall I not love you until the end of time
When the new day shall begin sublime
Will I not always love you most
Never to add up the cost
Are you not my lost cause
I shall not as your general pause
To engage from the rear
Through the flanks tear
Then face the obstacle
Of my loves debacle
Oh, how my love does drive me on
Ol scratch himself I must out-con
For the fight is with that old devil
Throwing good intentions against acts so evil
The fight shall remain on-going
As love for you I am showing
It is not time to say good-bye
Fow now is when I look into your lonely eye
Because love is to be found there
Of that I intend to have my share
I love you
So true
Would you please
let love not cease.

LETTERS TO LEIGH

Never the fool

We both have a notebook
In your own you said to look
In that I found more than one gentle expression
Also, your loves confession
Although they were for some other
Than your friend and brother
 I did not feel small
No, not at all
For I was quite happy
That you had written so sloppily
For when you wrote
To me a note
You would then be neat
Of love a feat
I know them all in my heart
For through them love did start
To inside me churn
Yes, to within me burn
Speaking plainly, it was quite a trip
Then to see each lip
Printed as a caper
On your note of paper
I have saved all of them
With one piece of film
Of you acting so cool
Never the fool
I am here yet not at the end
For I shall add to the love that I send.

LETTERS TO LEIGH

More letters of love to thee

These poems are yours
Because as I have told you before
I would lay down my life
To make you my wife
Add that cause to this other
I want to be your lover
Are there enough hours in the day
To say the things that I want to say
Not enough minutes in an hour
To fully feel loves power
Just not enough seconds in a minute
To take my love then on you pin it
Maybe there is a second to few in time
To grow dull on your love sublime
We are living life minute by minute
Should we not find some love in it
With our lives we could
Reject the bad and accept the good
Too often our self we lose
Then what we want often proves
That it is of short duration
Except in our situation
For I will keep writing until we have met
If that does not happen I shall write yet
More letters of love to thee
 perhaps you may one day see
 when I said that I love you
It was with a love that is true.

LETTERS TO LEIGH

This too is how I feel

I have told you everything
How I would buy for you a diamond ring
A house on the hill
With furs to feel
I know that you loved me then
I do know that you love me often
 I need not to know that you love me now
For love we did sow
Into each other
For one another
You said that you would love me always
Did not you say that your love stays
With me night and day
While I weep and when I play
Then you said that your love would stay
Never to go away
This to is how I too feel
Yet being without you is a bitter pill
I wonder how happy you are
Then has your hopes carried you far
I pray for you at every meal
When at night I on my knees kneel
Blessing Gods name
While praising his fame
As I ask will he do a little thing
Such as to me and you together bring
Tho if he does keep us apart
Please give to us happiness as an art.

LETTERS TO LEIGH

Being careful not to fall

If I seem depressed at any time
That does not show in my rhyme
I am just, I guess, all alone
Maybe because you never call on the phone
Hold I not your voice most precious
Would I not be most gracious
To from you hear
As my soul does tear
Love I not you above creation
Is not my love of long duration
Has it truly been months since we first met
For I still love you and yet
We have not words between us
Not joy, no love, nor kiss, without fuss
Is it just not everyday
That I ask God and pray
May you be safe and sound
For he does know where you are to be found
I do not have many words tonight
Yet I think of you then see the light
Then while my brain is still bright
To write to you is my delight
I now find that my eyes grow dim
As I hover near loves rim
Being careful not to fall
I will hang on then I shall
Have more words to send
May your love forever lend.

LETTERS TO LEIGH

I am calling day and night

Does forever mean forever
Never to sever
Such were the words used
When you spoke of our love that is true
I most heartily agreed
As I knelt on bended knee
You said that it would take time
To fix your life then be mine
My only worry
Is that you are sorry
That you said those things
As you wore my rings
Do you still love me enough
To change your life and be tough
To survive it all
Then still heed loves call
I am calling day and night
For I have seen loves light
Overcoming depth and height
To have you once more in my sight
Yet it is really still up to you
Tho I believe your heart to be blue
Without me your friend and brother
Who loves you as not another
Just walk outside your door
You I cannot ignore
Make a present of yourself
My pixie faced elf.

LETTERS TO LEIGH

If you are sad

Many hugs and kisses
To the one that my heart misses
I have missed you for so long
Ever do I miss your song
Beside me is where you do belong
While love beats loudly its gong
I cannot ignore
What I have said before
That I miss you like the earth misses rain
Like sorrow misses pain
If you are sad
You need to feel something bad
That would use
Or leave a soft emotional bruise
Then sooner or later
You begin to feel better
Yet your sorrow needs the pain
Because your heart does feel a sprain
That is part of the cure
Holding part of the lure
To come looking for salvation
For with love there is elation
This we need to hope for
While our hearts are sore
I know all of these things
For what they do not bring
Because I am missing a wife
Who is half of my life.

LETTERS TO LEIGH

I cannot be caught

Love is a slow moving train
From my heart to my brain
Covering over every hole
Within my soul
I may be on medication
Yet that does not stop my dedication
For from where you are
I do not want to be far
Cast away from your loving gaze
Even if there is a haze
Between us at present
I greatly resent
Anyone that has said
That our love is dead
I say yes, it is alive indeed
for yet my heart does bleed
What better proof
Than this simple truth
You are bone of my bone
Even when we are not alone
Always flesh of my flesh
For I am caught in the mesh
Of your net
Yet
I cannot be caught
For I have already been bought
By heaven
Then to you given.

LETTERS TO LEIGH

I need to hear your voice

I love you, I wish that you would call
Again in love I could then fall
Down onto my knees
There to give thanks to God then beg him please
Let you be mine
Right up to the end of time
That is as it should be
For I will love you through eternity
All stays so silent
My thoughts are quiet
I need to hear your voice
Yet I have not a choice
Only to listen to myself
Of the memories that you have left
Me from our brief affair
Especially of your hair
Also your face
Dressed in lace
Tho my favourite was that voice
Which never made noise
That I did not find
Except to bring peace of mind
I still have all of each piece
You are yet my golden fleece
Always are you my holy grail
Forever I am too close to fail
If God will aid and support
I shall win loves sport

LETTERS TO LEIGH

For I have to say

I should not have stopped writing of you
It does seem that I have lost that spontaneity
Now I have to stop then think
Again my mind has to blink
I am often baffled
For my thoughts are waffled
Yet I never stopped praying
That you would be saying
Forever you do love me
Just as I do thee
I have thought of you every day
Then my love once more down I lay
I have never given up hoping
That we might one day be eloping
Here and now these words do come dear
Then sometimes I fear
That I may run out
Of words for my fount
Tho I know that the troubles lie
In not looking toward you eye to eye
For so long
I have missed your song
Now I must move along
Even if I am wrong
For I have to say
What may allay
Words that do pay
Until after today.

LETTERS TO LEIGH

To prevent a tear

I miss you so very much
Your taste and that touch
Tho what I do miss most
Is the precious love that we have lost
I love you so much my dear
That I should have nothing to fear
Yet I fear that what I have lost
Is beyond my power to pay the cost
For not only have I lost my beautiful wife
I have lost much happiness in life
As I so strive then as I do toil
Toward I hope unhappiness to foil
Hoping that still I have a chance
To once again share your glance
If I am then patient
Maybe something below sleeping latent
Will softly within you stir
Leading you to activate a new affair
Where I would never leave
You alone to grieve
Only to always be there
To prevent a tear
From falling to the floor
As I walked out of the door
Then I would hold you only to myself
Until only love was left
Do you see that I miss you so much
I miss your taste and that soft touch.

LETTERS TO LEIGH

I have need to call

Why do not I just call or write
To make sure that everything is all right
Because I am waiting on that love of yours
To open the doors
That I then may be a friend
For that is what we arranged
Before I became deranged
With waiting
To hear your call that I am anticipating
You leave me not a choice
I must hear your voice
Is it only I that has to call
Either to stand or to fall
I shall call then find out
If I will give a shout
Or if I shall keep waiting
Anticipating
Our eventually
Finding ecstasy
With one another
For each other
It only does take one call
To either win or lose all
I must wait until when
You are ready then
If I call you at the right time
Happiness will be mine

LETTERS TO LEIGH

My love is as strong

I love you most truly
Do not treat me so cruelly
Just give me a chance
With our romance
It is true that I am far away
Yet I have much to say
That you are beautiful, for instance
Then would you like to dance
I love you too much my dear
To have you shed your tear
The love that I feel for you is just enough
For me to keep from playing rough
As the sun does go from east to west
I love you all of that time and the rest
Of the night
It is my delight
To fashion for your fame
These words so hard to tame
For to love you is my fate
Yes I love you and cannot hate
Did you not heal my broken spirit
Then touch my heart so that I still feel it
Perhaps if I lost my love for you
Bad things I would then spew
Yet there is not a worry
Or need to be sorry
For my love is as strong
As our separation is long.

LETTERS TO LEIGH

Out of reach, like a dove

I need an opening line
To make a rhyme
I need someone to love
From my hearts hidden cove
Love is best if it is shown
For someone that I have known
Who I could name
Yet could not tame
Whose love in return
I would not spurn
She does not have to be a lady
Just a woman, a friend maybe
Already I do know someone
Who does fit these traits every one
How she is so far above
Out of reach like a dove
Although she might disown
Remain does she all alone
Because to her I am
In soul a twin of Siam
She must feel as much
As I do without her touch
I see now
Just how
That I lost
At such cost
To her and myself
Fleeting mental health.

LETTERS TO LEIGH

When I am so far away

It is time to write again
To my special friend
Who does help me through each day
Then gladly helps me to find the way
Just her memory
Is a lamp for me
When I am in danger of falling
Her voice yet always does come calling
Guiding me on
Back toward home
I love her for this
Also for bringing me bliss
When I am so far away
I am still under her sway
A taskmaster so pleasant
Shall I not be forever her peasant
Working in the love field
Baring my heart without a shield
Anytime she may choose
Always she may have me to use
As long as she does not send me away
From under her sway
I shall work hard and long
To again hear her song
In love I am her slave
Anytime she could save
For if she would spare the whip
 then may love slip.

LETTERS TO LEIGH

To a cherished place

Is my love so short
Would it hold up in court
Do I need a defence
For a love that is so immense
I have loved you from
The first moment on
Ever from the first time that you spoke
Love in me has awoke
When you grinned
I then felt love again
When for the first time that you cried
The love in me tried
To calm the commotion
With balm of love lotion
 when your eye was less wetter
We then both felt better
My brain is allowed
To keep some things hallowed
Yet love has gained entry
Past my minds sentry
To a cherished place
Near unto my souls vase
May unworthy thoughts cease
Stay worthy thoughts that please
For God may allow you near
Without too much fear
We shall work out loves quirk
For that is how love does work.

LETTERS TO LEIGH

For the love that I hold

If I have not said that I love you before
Now I am saying that I just adore
You and yourself
A very special elf
If I could write down
The love that I own
I would have many a scroll
For the love that I hold
That is overflowing
Which now is showing
In a little way
Everyday
Now I am praying
That you will be saying
Ever you love me so
Then with me you will go
To make a happy home
Where never will my love be alone
For we shall have each other
To love one another
That is my hope with my dream
To live on life's cream
You are the gentle vessel
For which I must wrestle
Being so careful not to break
That love which I would gently take
Now I am ready for a new scroll
For my love has grown bold.

LETTERS TO LEIGH

We feel bold

There is a calm before the storm
When we must all feel forlorn
Kind of hopeless, kind of helpless
Kind of out of place
It does seem that life
With all of its strife
May bring us down
To the ground
While lightning shafts flash asunder
as the thunder so cold does thunder
We feel bold
In our humble abode
To there make light of such a night
For tis part of the human condition
To be at odds with perdition
Because when the chips are down
We may wear a frown
Yet all are making haste
To have a taste
Of the whole that life does offer
Both the rich and the pauper
So when you see storm clouds approaching
Know then that pleasure you will soon be
poaching
For as the lightning is ever brightened
Your joy will be enlightened
While as the storm begins to rumble
The shallow part of man again does crumble.

LETTERS TO LEIGH

I just have to see

I am supposed to be patient
With this love that is latent
Waiting for the time
When you do read this rhyme
I hope that these words make you happy
That it is not too shabby
For you know that I do love you
That is I love so true
You have said that you love me so
That love is not cruel I know
 your voice does lay about me little short of a
caress
Just your touch on me does bless
I will wait on you until the grass turns blue
For you must know that I am in love with you
I love you my darling
There is not a need to be quarrelling
When we are joined as man and wife
Ever forever shall we have a love filled life
I will kiss you good morn
Never to leave you forlorn
We shall wake up the moon
Then breakfast at noon
I will confess my love before all men
Then to God I shall confess my sin
So that our days will prove
To be in loves grove
I just have to see
Where to our love shall lead.

LETTERS TO LEIGH

Yet your love was laying there

This medicine is stealing my thoughts
For you of them I have fought
Trying to save a few
For me and you
My tears for you I have shed
As this heart for you has bled
My own soul for you has also cried
For I cannot ransom you from my mind
I too have a daily routine
While you are at your washing machine
Now I am learning how to socialize
For I had poor skills I now realize
Maybe that had something to do
With the way that I did woo
Yet your love was laying there
I only tried to take it somewhere
from you I took a large drink
Then into love began to sink
Up until now
It still does flow
As I have yet to say my prayers
For I am trying to climb heavens stairs
With a message to love
Residing up above
To please come to my aid
Devotedly you may be paid
Tho if you hesitate
Still my payment will not be late.

LETTERS TO LEIGH

Of you I thought

I am trying to find you among my thoughts
I thought you lost then sought
For you my precious
With love of the freshest
All for my princess
Because of her dances
That she had for me last night
Until morning bright
Ended our affair
Of dancing in air
By being awoken
With a word that was spoken
Saying, get up,
I said, I need my love cup
Whereby love I do sup,
Then I stepped out of bed
As I shook my head
To clear away the cobwebs
From their dusty shed
Of you I thought
You who I have sought
Sleeping
Then awakening
While my trivial chores I neglect
Yet I must win your respect
How better than to do
As I softly woo
While I write of love to you.

To build into her a flame

What may you do about it
You are there and here I sit
I will love you all that I dare
Then even call it a love affair
I have loved you as much as I wanted
For your silence has left me undaunted
You I have with me every day
Because I love you in every way
Are not you with me when down I do lie
You are with me when I sigh
For I love to give forth
On how much to me you are worth
Yes, I never make sport
When it does come to my love fort
Here muffled is my silence
For my heart does remain in alliance
With the queen of my heart
There I hope love will start
To build into her a flame
That only I may tame
Then as she gathers steam
I shall hope that she has seen
That I am only the fellow
Who may make her nice and mellow
I am standing at her door
My knock I hope she does not ignore
If she opens with a little kindness
She will find much happiness.

LETTERS TO LEIGH

On making it into heaven

Jesus came to earth to save men
By dying on the cross he gave heaven
To those who would seek
Through a world that is bleak
Jesus was God and son of God
Yet at his fathers nod
He was hung on the cross
To save mankind's dross
Now Jesus is high priest
Our prayers must pass through his wrist
Before the father they reach
Whose answers or silence teach
Us to be God fearing men
Though susceptible to sin
Therefore we have his word
Which cuts at sin as a sword
Jesus became a man
I am just as I am
Yet what Jesus could do
I should try to do too
The odds are even
On making it into heaven
If we just live the life
Free from strife
Love our fellow
While evil swallow
One day he shall call
then on my knees I will fall.

Some peace of mind

It is terrible to be afraid
After everything has been said
You are still afraid
The fear is not allayed
No where to run, no where to hide
Your fear is always at your side
If you look for help from friends
Maybe they will take you in
Surely soon they will begin
To use your fear again
What about your family
Dare to risk another calamity
Family do not always listen
To a tale that makes your face glisten
Should you tell it to your priest
He will answer with words that are chaste
Well, who do you tell
In this paranoid hell
Tell anyone that you trust
Then again until you bust
Talk to family and friends
Then continue on this trend
For one day you will find
Some peace of mind
Maybe you will not only hear
That inner fear
Then you may face the terrible
With a mind that is sensible.

LETTERS TO LEIGH

Waiting to be felled

Now that I have
Our love to save
Please do not lay blame
If I do give our love fame
From the highest mountain
Let loves fountain
Tumble
Rumble
Along
With its song
Plainly
To the sea
Let loves freedom ring
For the truth that it does bring
Will set us free
Like a tree
Left alone
In forest gloom
Waiting to be felled
For loves knell
With a mighty noise
Loves great voice
Rings out loud and clear
An example of our love, dear
Let our love be known
Let our love be shown
With our love let there be renown
With our love we have flown.

LETTERS TO LEIGH

Yet you do still hold sway

Was I scared
Or afraid
Of love growing
Were you knowing
That I was not
For love has not
Made me afraid
Of what has yet been said
Which is that we love each other
Also as sister and brother
For how could love ever be
If I did not set you free
For I have it all
To save you from a fall
I am watching you inside of my head
How your eyes do grow moist and red
When things are not going right
 I do wish for you to gain your sight
Then find your light
To help you through the night
Because I am now far away
Yet you do still hold sway
Over my being
For I am not leaving this place
Except to face
Finding
You whose love is binding.

LETTERS TO LEIGH

For love has not forsook

The law of love
Came from above
It says to love each other
As sister and brother
Yes, that is a good law
As we have all saw
While we were growing up
On love to sup
Then we meet somebody
Who may treat us shoddy
Then little by little
We forget loves riddle
Until we are filled with lies
Then other vice
Until we defiantly
Come to our eventuality
A living death
At our own behest
Yet there is the way that is good
Just as it should
Be for all who look
For love has not forsook
Those that have tasted
Have not wasted
Because at the end of their days
Is the way
That does lead to life
Seeking away from needless strife.

To be cheerful

How far may love go
Do you know
Perhaps it is past
Maybe love shall last
Who does know
Or may show
Us whether if a year from now
We may take a bow
That is a chance
Which we must balance
In loves scale
For we cannot fail
If we are sure of care
While full of cheer
Through life's each up then down
With side-steps thrown
At us now and then
Yet we need only grin
For together shall we make it thru
Tho life is cruel
Then our love so good
Will guide us to where it should
Then we may float along
With your song
Until we arrive
At loves hive
Then all of the bees
Shall make love for thee.

LETTERS TO LEIGH

Near or far away

In two or three days
Our love may play
Yet for now
Love may plan anyhow
How shall we meet
Then will with love treat
Each other
As lover or sister and brother
Be that as it may
We should allow our love to play
As await we then that wonderful day
Near or far away
We may be a child again
You shall be my special friend
Will I not you try to entertain
As I make my love for you so plain
With all of my time of you I do think
Yet I do not need to sink
Into depression
While I make my love confession
You will forever be the only one
Where to me the seeds of love are sown
I shall wait for them to grow
Then find the flower that they show
I will take a little scent
For that is what on my love has been spent
Then I shall take a little more
For the fruit of your love I do adore.

LETTERS TO LEIGH

Your hearts tender fruit

I feel that we are old friends
Should not we hope to continue on this trend
For it is my delight
To keep you feeling bright
If I may, that is,
I will bring to you bliss
Then if I do
We shall call it woo
Forever if you make it through
I will marry you
That is my goal
With saving my soul
I do give it great import
Of that I make not sport
Now I know your style
 that you are in denial
Yet from that I may coax
Without using a hoax
Your love toward my way
Where it will stay
To mine adjacent
As long as I am patient
Not to bruise
Or misuse
Your hearts tender fruit
Like a brute
I am not
Of your love soon to have forgot.

Learn to live again

Let me lay you down
In your gown
Place within mine your hand
Instead of my wand
Poetry we may make
Love does not have to be fake
I will not want to let you go
Before you believe then know
That I love you with my soul
Only you may make it whole
If you add yours
Before the hour
Is up
Then we may sup
From loves cup
As like a pup
We shall be frisky
At something so risky
As this love
From above
Then there will be a trace
On our face
Of a tear
Yet not fear
We shall begin
To have a grin
Then
Learn to live again.

LETTERS TO LEIGH

That does not ever leave me all alone

I cannot change the world
I merely stand with banners unfurled
Nor may I change the way
People act from day-to-day
I am only one man
Who some seek to ban
From their bad kingdom
Which I would fling-down
Except that I am seeking
Your love to be sneaking
That love is the true one
That does not ever leave me all alone
I love you more than I may tell
You pull me through each little hell
From you not hearing
While for your love I am swearing
Is mine to possess
If I use finesse
In a few months more
I may have you to adore
I love you so much
Forever I miss your touch
Miss I that voice
With all of your noise
I hope that you do not miss
Your chance to read this
For this only does mean
You are my queen.

LETTERS TO LEIGH

In finding you

I will find love through the fog
Between the trees moss then over log
Shall I find love that is right
By the star shining bright
I will not be brought to an impasse
By my hearts compass
My feet will be true
In finding you
I love you so much
So much I miss your touch
I long to feel your lip
Then from therein take a sip
 to climb upon that mountain
To find again loves fountain
I will find you where you are
Where you are I do not care
Shall I not bring you to our home
For us to be alone
May you have what you want
I will just hang around and haunt
Your heart
Until love does start
To build a flame
For my name
Then you say yes
To my embrace
For we shall be one
Tho with love alone.

LETTERS TO LEIGH

The many ways

What should we do
About our love that is true
It is becoming lonely
Being an only
Son in our affair
Yet I miss your stare
Need I not to feel your touch
For it is nice and such
A pleasant thing
For you to bring
I need to kiss your lip
Then take a sip
While with loves cup
I shall take a sup
Into loves fount
I will count
The many ways
That your love does make me to delay
For you I am waiting
Anticipating
Appreciating
Our dating
That is to come
When you come home
With your song
To where you belong
A nice home I shall fix
For there shall live Mrs. Nix.

LETTERS TO LEIGH

To follow the flame

A silent flame
Wherein not shame
Is love
From above
I pick up an ember
Then become a member
That is love
With its gentle shove
Love guides me in the right direction
Without my prediction
Of where I am going
I am only knowing
That when I come there
Your love shall I share
All of my critics aside
I will this love ride
Until we are no longer apart
Then we may start
The flame a little higher
To make love a little shyer
Then somehow make love more precious
For love does make me more tenacious
To follow the flame
Then take aim
With all of my art
A love quenching dart
Tho not to put the flame out
Of my love fount.

LETTERS TO LEIGH

Even if there is not a song

My words are coming a little better
Now that I realize there will not be a letter
For I must carry on
Even if there is not a song
Then should you one day read this
I hope that you find some special bliss
For now I must write anyway
Because it does help me to pass each day
I am not angry, I try not to be sad
I only wish that I had
More time to spend
With my heart to lend
On this kind of day
When you need me in a special way
As I have said before
I shall keep turning the pages of this lore
For that does help me
Then deep down I believe
That one day you will read this
While thinking maybe then offer up a kiss
For my writing that is enough of a reason
That I will keep doing so through loves season
You have never turned my love letters down
Have only once made me frown
Yet time does ease all pain
Truly it is sunny after the rain
If we are patient he may show
Us a miracle in a rainbow.

LETTERS TO LEIGH

Upon loves good fruit

There is not any hard evidence
Or lack of good sense
In this case
Of love erased
Yet in my heart it is chiselled
For my heart has received a missile
To go on loving thee
As I have always loved ye
Through the past
For it will last
Up to the day
When we shall play
Jump and shout
Happily all about
That we are together again
Then we may be as one, friend
On that day
We may say
That we have been through it all
Yet heard we loves call
For us to be together
To be separated never
Then one day we will be
Sitting underneath loves tree
In the good shade
That our love has made
Then we shall place a tooth
Upon loves good fruit.

LETTERS TO LEIGH

As I go through life

That first kiss
Was great, not less
For it opened my loving eye
To the wide sky
Which had been empty before
Yet now held beauty galore
That first kiss
Did all of this
It has kept me so happy through the day
That I cannot count each and every way
That it has kept me from feeling low
When life is just too slow
I know not what I would do
If I had not you to woo
For you are the one and only
That does keep me from being lonely
Only you are my star set into the sky
From where I guide my ship by
As I go through life
You relieve the strife
Forever you are making me to ask God please
Then you are there to help me sleep with ease
When I find myself upon my knees
You do help the troubled waters to cease
Then forever to keep me on my toes
Looking for where lives water does flow
That first kiss
Did all of this.

LETTERS TO LEIGH

Holding her by her glove

Of love I have had a taste
Not one drop did I waste
I would come back more
To this love store
Only for that I am too poor
To unlock the door
I must wait on it to open
By someone else hoping
To drink the dew
Meant for the few
I had to drink hurriedly
For I had not a key
Yet I kept on watch
For someone to open the latch
Then drop their key
Should I not pick it up in a hurry
If so, I would not put it within my pocket
For then I could put it into the locket
Soon to give the door a shove
For I may then help myself to love
There I would be at any odd hour
To pick from an assortment for love a flower
Then I would come to my nightly roost
As our love would give me a boost
Up the steps to loves door
Even tho once I had been poor
I now have her love
Holding her by her glove.

LETTERS TO LEIGH

You want to put the fire out

Love burns a silent fire
Living on its desire
To join another flame
So the greater, may be the same
With each other
As sister and brother
Or lover
Then each cover
In their haste
To have a taste
Of each others flame
Which is the same
For one as the other
Knowing that they must not smother
Their fuel
Which would be cruel
When they should
Ignite loves wood
To bring about
A fiery fount
Of little flames
That they may claim
Then the fire would spread
Upon our heads
To cover ourselves
With fiery elves
Until with your mouth
You want to put the fire out.

LETTERS TO LEIGH

My heart yet demanding

I just wanted to write a poem
Like finding a rare coin
Of my esteem it would be a token
About what between us was bespoken
Back in April and may
As we had a merry-round-de-lay
Whether or not were you mine
Or mine yet to find
Then like musical chairs
The music ended the sweet flair
Tho I was left standing
My heart yet demanding
A place to be still
To there at your feet kneel
Then you said to keep the token
Of what was bespoken
Between just us
No lust to cuss
I would like to tip fortune
Into the way that I am searching
For love is what I am looking for
There I hope that it is near the door
That opens up to life
Which does lead away from strife
I hope that I shall find you there
With your beautiful stare
So precious to my sight
To welcome into the light.

LETTERS TO LEIGH

Down my love do I lay

Come with me back to may
When love did have that way
Again, let us not be late
To relive our loves fate
Like a moth that cannot find the way
I have not had enough to say
May I not tell you that I love you enough
To be silent is too tough
Within my brain
Then I refrain
From making an addition
To the sedition
Presently in you engaged
Over why may not I have
You with my bath
For I have been doing
So much wooing
Since you I met
Cannot you let
Your love meet mine half-way
Where it is sure to stay
Out of trouble
Then love may bubble
Up with joy
To be near your boy
 then shall it be for me to say
Down my love do I lay.

LETTERS TO LEIGH

Onto loves garden

Cast thy love before
Me once more
The love that I adore
That does make my heart soar
Above the clouds with joy
Turn my heart into a toy
A mere plaything
For you a trifling
For you do make love happen
Even when you are napping
With love you are soaked through
 I must taste your brew
Then while I am drunk
Your love has not shrunk
Instead it has grew
Like I knew
Good love always
Does multiply the ways
For us to love each other
With love for one another
The good seed of love
Fell from above
Onto loves garden
Which was full of pardon
May I pick one
Because of the error that I have done
I might take two
For I have done a few.

LETTERS TO LEIGH

If that is to be

I would give up my gun
Then all of my other fun
For just one more good-bye
Just one more should I
Tell you that my love is true
In love I am with you
Is what I would reply
That twould be not a lie
Yet small credit that does me now
When I have lost you somehow
Not to anything that I could have done
Nor to anything that I could have won
You were won away by your child
So tender, meek, and mild
What chance did I to dare
Except your life to share
I made my offer fair and square
With my open heart laid bare
You did not say no, nor did you say yes
Yet you could not add any to my bliss
Tho you took me aside
To there where you cried and cried
Saying, this is how it must be for now
Yet I know that the Lord will bring us together
somehow,
If that is to be
Then we shall know that we
Will be together to the end
Along with the love that the Lord sends.

LETTERS TO LEIGH

A love dew delicious

My words may seem a mere trifle
Yet my love is beautiful
Of all of my treasure
My love is without measure
Also it would give me pleasure
If you had it at your leisure
Throughout your days
Then to let my love become a maze
Through that for you to find your way
In that for you to stay
Are you not one of the Lords blessings
That I am to be kissing
For I discard none
Of the Lords gifts, not one
Is a trifle
Or something to stifle
Yet each does gain attention
When I make mention
Of them in my prayers
As I do the love that is ours
I know that God does listen
When my forehead must glisten
For he may give what I ask
After I finish some task
Yet my point is that you are precious
A love dew delicious
When again I am king
For your love I shall ring.

LETTERS TO LEIGH

In my hand until warm

I do not know much about poetry
I am hoping some is coming from me
I do not know much about poetry
I just hope that my words do be
I do not know much about poetry
Yet it does exist within my fancy
I have never read much poetry
Yet now its worth I may see
I have never read much poetry
Nor ever had much read to me
I have never written much poetry
Yet I am working on a volume of fifty
I have never written much poetry
Yet I may write one shortly
I have never written much poetry
Yet now and then I try
I do not know much about love
Except that I would hold it like a velvet glove
In my hand until warm
Then your heart I would disarm
Your heart to mine then I would join
As I feel my love stir in my loin
A poet I cannot claim to be
Yet your love I am able to set free
I am not a poet and I am not lying
Barely do I make a rhyme.

LETTERS TO LEIGH

A special situation

It is not my fancy clothes
Nor rings that show
That I have a style
That does drive my share wild
It is not my silly locks
Nor my special socks
That must knock them out
My love fount
It just seems that they know
About loves whose who
For they are able to tell
That my heart is not for sale
Yet to lend
To a friend
Is an everyday trend
Then I bend
Over to help any special one
I do know them by their overall tone
For I like some for the way that they talk
I like some for the way that they walk
A special situation
Needs not an explanation
Yet I just only need a special friend
With a willing heart to lend
You should know that her looks would be true
Reminding me of you
I almost think that you would like me
To find someone then make love beautifully.

LETTERS TO LEIGH

All here safe and sound

If you find yourself again
Separated from your friend
Have a little faith and a little hope
With a little love so that you may cope
For when you meet once more
You may each adore
Having found again
Your lost friend
Yet if your paths never meet
Ever where finding that you miss that friend so
sweet
Send your prayers to God above
On the wings of a snow white dove
For as your path does wind around
Someday you may hear the sound
Of an old familiar voice
Standing out above the noise
There fall at once unto your knees
Asking God please o please
Do not now tease
Let me find that she's
All here safe and sound
Was lost yet now is found
We shall feel glory bound
Now that I have come around
To take her by the hand
Then will we walk across the land
Shall we to love forever stay close together
For we have chosen to be tethered.

LETTERS TO LEIGH

Then love moved into my vein

It is allowed for a poet to say that he loves you
Even if he does not in a way it is still true
So let me write rightly
Yet you take it lightly
Do not become sad
Become neither sore nor mad
If I say that I love you
I really, really do
For the poetry of my brain
Will keep our friendship unstrained
If you understand this
You may find a little bliss
In these words that I am using
If your ego I am not bruising
Now that the above is out of the way
I would like to say
That I love you a lot
Also that you have a special spot
A special place
Within a special space
Inside of my heart
Where my love did start
To act
With tact
When you came onto the scene
Then love moved into my vein
As long as you stay
I shall love you with my word play.

LETTERS TO LEIGH

Dare you to enter glory's portal

No one my poems may touch
There is not one that is good enough
As I look around
For a model with a special sound
None may understand
What it is to be honoured with the pen
If I do not find one soon
I shall give myself a boon
Then write of you like a thief
Just to find some relief
She only has to be special
To me she must appeal
Yet I must keep writing
Even if her I am not sighting
Consider yourself, for example
I have already shown a sample
Of what is in my brain
Even yet now you keep on delaying
Tho I do not blame you, you are so busy
It is the other candidates that make me dizzy
I just cannot come out and ask them
Would you like to participate in my sham
Do you want your name to be immortal
Dare you to enter glories portal
I am not even asking for sex
It is my mind that I must flex
Do not introduce me to a friend
A poet and model must be special kin.

LETTERS TO LEIGH

Waiting, waiting to catch her eye

I would like to be alone with love
Like a power line with a dove
I should not know what to say
Or if I could anyway
I would touch her there on the shoulder
According to her eyes I may grow bolder
Yet I would be happy just to sit
 to then allow my broken heart to knit
I would not engage in conversation
For would I not be involved with love conservation
My heart would be one full sigh
Waiting, waiting to catch her eye
All that I should need would be to sit near
While I practice to myself calling her dear
Then it would be heaven to hold her hand
If things could follow an unlaid plan
Maybe she would take a hint
Adding to the colour of my eyes tint
It would be my fondest hope
If with our feelings we could cope
Until I had the nerve
To give toward love a serve
Then if she took my meaning
With love I would be preening
There is something that I need to say
To break the ice anyway
How about, it is a beautiful night,
Have you ever seen such a sight.

LETTERS TO LEIGH

With the words that I have woven

It has been more than one week
Since my book of Leigh has peeked
I do not know how to say this
Only that, I just miss her with the bliss
That I had from writing
creating
A thing so beautiful
Compared to my life which is dull
Her love I cannot betray
Yet I must write anyway
Her I cannot forget
Yet
Her I must place
Inside of my heart as a safe place
Then there she must dwell
While our love is ill
To others I must move on
To hear them sing their song
I want her most
Yet she is beyond my cost
Still to her honour
I do pledge my armour
She may meet that and cheer
Or with only a sneer
My love I have proven
With the words that I have woven
I now feel secure
To stop another's tear.

LETTERS TO LEIGH

Into loves cup

I hold my dreams in my hand
Like footsteps in the sand
As I am walking about the land
For someone to hold my hand
Of love I am looking for traces
Yet I have been to all of the wrong places
Until I touched thy hand
Then I picked up my wand
Promising my love
Hidden within my secret cove
For you I would like to come to know
Maybe love for me you would gently show
I felt love for you from the start
Right from my heart
Please do not take apart
Then put into your cart
To take home
Where you are alone
It is made to use
Not to lose
Myself I would like to introduce
Then your shoes I could unloose
Something says that you like me
Then that does say that you are she
Who may lift me up
Into loves cup
With a little sugar and crème
Placing love in between.

LETTERS TO LEIGH

I am always asking

At times love is fast and loud
Yet sometimes like a slow cloud
All nice and quiet
With mist that are white
Providing shade
Where it is then bade
From up above
The purest love
In it I find satisfaction
While I make my love extraction
Yet when it is passing
I am always asking
Why cannot there be more
For a heart that is sore
I will find the answer
To this humble banter
By looking to another
If I may find any other
To replace what I have lost
Then to repay the cost
Of playing the game
With the stakes the same
I do not offer any blame
Only to make it my aim
To shake, roll, and rattle
In my next love battle
What love I did gain
Does make loves next battle plain.

LETTERS TO LEIGH

I needed to help her out

I hardly know her yet
Tho I am able to tell that her eyes stay wet
Over something in her life
Creating for her strife
She was sitting at a table
Looking like she was right out of a fable
With long brown hair
Lonely green eyes for her stare
She knew my name
Of her I knew the same
She could tell from my looks
That I had felt hard knocks
I knew her reputation
Also her situation
Which was not as good
As it should
Have been
For someone I called friend
I needed to help her out
To help soften her pout
Though she wore a grin
I saw through that again
In a way round-a-bout
Am I, I am going to ask her out
Then we may go to a park
To listen if love should hark
If it would do so
The halves of our heart will woo.

LETTERS TO LEIGH

I received that love for free

It is not an easy chore
To continue loves lore
After I have done
What went before
Yet she would understand
That I am a love needing man
I do not dim her flame
By my new aim
Which is to ignite fire
Into those hearts that are tired
She must not mind
If others I find
In need of the power
Of loves shower
Tho even if she does
Then if her heart is all a-buzz
I must still do
What I have to
For me to woo
Anew
Broken heart
I shall take the broken part
Along with love lotion
Then adding loves motion
Heal the damage there-in
With my love medicine
I received that love for free
For love there is not a fee.

LETTERS TO LEIGH

When upon me you shed loves dew

I did tell you that I would write
Before the passing of the night
I would like to tell
Where my love has fell
Why did I not pick it up
Because I wished for it to sup
At the root
From the offshoot
Of the tree of your love
Still growing high above
The moss where my love did lay
Would I not leave it until the day
When upon me you shed loves dew
That I may again live to woo
Then I picked my love up from off of the ground
For new love within myself I had found
Saying give to me love please
I fell onto my knees
To thank thee
For thy attention on me
I let my love come all inside
Even though I had not a bride
She had given me one thing
Of that love I now sing
For maybe one day soon
Love may grant a boon
Then handing me the pleasure and strife
Giving to me my own wife.

LETTERS TO LEIGH

Feel free to take my love

Feel free to love
Give others a gentle shove
Feel free to touch
Yet never say ouch
Feel free to talk
Please do not sulk
Feel free to look
Then read me like a book
Feel free to give your heart
I will not take it apart
Feel free to wink
Then into love to sink
Feel free to smile
So as to leave your denial
Feel free to kiss
That-that you miss
Feel free to be a friend
Then may your heart mend
Feel free to relax
So as to feel love to the max
Feel love once more
Then your heart will not be sore
Feel my love for you
As we begin to woo
Feel your heart unloose
To cure it of its bruise
Feel free to take my love
To within your hidden cove.

LETTERS TO LEIGH

The same in fears

I long to feel your touch
May it heal my ouch
You I do not know
Yet I do want love to show
Us both
The truth
About love
Then to us give a gentle shove
Into ecstasy
Tho not recklessly
I think that you may be able to tell
That I am in a gentle hell
Do I say to you how
That I feel sweet love for you now
Or do I wait
To anticipate
The surprise
In your eyes
As I speak the word
That could then for your heart cure
I am not even where
You are
For you are there
Yet I am here
Apart in years
Yet the same in fears
We shall get it together
Love will find shelter.

LETTERS TO LEIGH

Just me and you

You hold my love in the palm of your hand
If I fail my tears will outnumber all of the grains of
sand
I am a believer of love at first sight
For now I may say that I have seen the light
N the past my tears have overran my palms
While my mind was filled with psalms
I loved her yet she did not appreciate
Being near to loves gate
Love is such a wonderful free gift
There is not a need to be a thrift
Come one, come all
There is plenty and love shall
Find those
Who know
That something so free
Was meant for you and me
Yet please do not delay
For there is love to pay
When we stand near
Without our common fear
Just me and you
With nothing to lose
Except our pain
With nothing to gain
Except everything
Then to bring
Words of love
From within our hidden cove.

LETTERS TO LEIGH

Into love that is true

You do not know it
Yet I am your poet
It is my job
To find words to rob
Which describe you
In a way that is true
It is a job that is wonderful
you are so beautiful
Just a little shy
With a dislike of lies
To make things easy
You could be sleazy
Yet you are not
For you are pretty hot
Just be yourself
In good health
I shall find the way
To make love pay
Tribute to your beauty
Because that is my duty
You do not have to wonder how
Only come out then take your bow
I am your poet
You must know it
As a woman of class
I will help you to pass
Through
Into love that is true.

LETTERS TO LEIGH

After I give to you a gentle shove

It is out of deep respect
That your love I do expect
I give to you in return
Love that you should not spurn
I know that I am not so attractive
As to make your love reactive
Yet if a pure heart you do want
Take mine then vaunt
Yourself high upon love
after I give to you a gentle shove
I will bring you down a little slow
Yet never as low
As you were
Before I came here
I just want to get
To know you then let
Two interesting ones
Have a little fun
I cannot hardly wait
Until you reach that state
Of being yourself
While loving my stealth
The day is coming soon
At loves high noon
When there will be a test
Over who is best
With their pen
Along with their heart open.

LETTERS TO LEIGH

These thoughts of love I am thinking

I need someone for my new book
Someone with a special look
I think that you may help to fill the role
While in so doing help me to heal my soul
We have not known each other for long
Tho I bet that you have a special song
As long as this pen I make play
You may sing your round-de-lay
I strongly urge
That you allow love to surge
Over the surf
Onto loves turf
I have love that is true
I shall be gentle and not hurt you
Where else may you find love so good
Or elsewhere would love be as it should
We are two hearts
For now apart
Yet they may be one
If we let them join
These thoughts of love I am thinking
When I think of you I am not blinking
From the lights inside of my head
Over what I should have said
What I put down here
I am willing to share
Like my hope
That with love you may ever cope.

LETTERS TO LEIGH

Please do not feel bad

I do not recall know what to write
Only that I do know that it was a welcome sight
Then quite
A delight
For you to put up such might
In your fight
To turn me down
Yet then you turned me on
With your acceptance
Without reluctance
To take my book
Then to have a look
Inside
Beside
All of the thoughts
That I had fought
To make me ask
You to do that task
I threw to you a curve
You then returned a serve
I took a swing
Then made the bell ring
I love you enough
To make it tough
Please do not feel bad
If you wish that you had
Let it pass
Around that heart, my lass.

LETTERS TO LEIGH

I am a friend that is true

I have not really had a chance
To take your love for a dance
Yet if I ever do
I shall begin to woo
You over to my side
While I wait on the tide
To pull your heart
Like it pulled mine apart
We do not really know one another
We are still sister and brother
Tho all of that does hang
On a minutes change
I love you and I love to write
Do not I welcome your love on sight
You have had, I know, a tough past
Yet this new love is meant to last
I have never seen you without your smile
I love, I know, that style
You always have a pleasant tongue
That does soak up thanks like a sponge
If I am not in love with you
I am a friend that is true
For if our love does last
Love shall cast
Along with lend
To us being friends
A many coloured blanket
Whereupon we shall dine on loves banquet.

LETTERS TO LEIGH

If you cannot see

Time is not getting me anywhere
I must write about you, I swear
I thought that I would wait
Then move at your gait
Yet at this stage of the game
I must not reveal your name
For it is my hope
That you may cope
With my moving along
Without your song
I must continue my mission
Without your permission
For it is my duty
To honour your beauty
Even if I have not asked
Your opinion in this talk
We do not seem to talk much
Never do we touch
Yet I have the feeling
That you are in need of emotional healing
I want to get
To know you yet
If you cannot see
Just make believe
That I may be that friend
When troubles seem to never have an end
I want to write a book
revealing you and your look.

LETTERS TO LEIGH

A way to stay in love

I do not know your history
Yet your future will be a love story
With you in sight
I shall write
Words that will be sweet balm
Upon my palms
I shall tickle your ears
With sweet words to hear
Your future
Will be sure
Then secure
In Lamore
Beginning with your eyes unstained
I will gaze at hair so brownish sheen
Never would I like to see you without your smile
For you have it all the while
Everywhere that I go
Your smile is there I know
I do not write this in jest
I want to be your artist
Putting down on paper
The things of you that do caper
In my sight
By your light
I have lost her who I cannot replace
Yet with you I may trace
A way to stay in love
With the one who I gave the gloves.

LETTERS TO LEIGH

While I stood ready for her call

I wish for you the love that I first knew
The same true love that I blew
Her hand, I wish, was in my palm
As she sang her psalm
I wish for the day that we first met
When she gave to me a cigarette
The smoke filled the air
As did the love of our affair
We did not meet in the best of places
Yet our love grew by paces
That matched the love that we bore
For one another and even more
There we tasted each other
Knew we then that we were sister and brother
Yet it was not a sin
For love to be in
For she gave to me all
While I stood ready for her call
That she would use
When she was afraid that me she would lose
Our love was as mad as mad could be
Yet she was never mad at me
Our love was faster than fast
Forever was it meant to last
Until the devil entered the scene
Then acted he toward me so mean
For he took my love away
Down to this very day.

LETTERS TO LEIGH

While I stood ready for her call

I wish for you the love that I first knew
The same true love that I blew
Her hand, I wish, was in my palm
As she sang her psalm
I wish for the day that we first met
When she gave to me a cigarette
The smoke filled the air
As did the love of our affair
We did not meet in the best of places
Yet our love grew by paces
That matched the love that we bore
For one another and even more
There we tasted each other
Knew we then that we were sister and brother
Yet it was not a sin
For love to be in
For she gave to me all
While I stood ready for her call
That she would use
When she was afraid that me she would lose
Our love was as mad as mad could be
Yet she was never mad at me
Our love was faster than fast
Forever was it meant to last
Until the devil entered the scene
Then acted he toward me so mean
For he took my love away
Down to this very day.

LETTERS TO LEIGH

Loves loosening coil

This is what I do for a living, I use my head
Not to listen to what others have said
Or that which has been read
To this I have been bred
Until down the path I have led
You as my wife to be wed
Until my love has then fled
To be with you in our bed
For you I cannot get over
Please come share my cover
Come, please, near and hover
Forever, come be my lover
I shall disarm you gently
Then feel your love so simply
In that I would bathe
When my heart turns on your lathe
Until you I do render
Pure love as a cinder
While my juices boil
As you turn
To toil
You shall churn
Yet will not soil
Then shall you love learn
That you will not foil
Loves loosening coil
To find a better grip
Before love has time to slip.

Loving everything

Is it medicine time
I am glad that mine is fine
Give me a double dose
That this love-cold I may lose
Then love so pure will I breathe
While pure love I shall bequeath
To all of those standing around
Who does hear the sound
Of pure love being felt
That true love being helt
For all of us
Without a fuss
Nor to-do
Not ever with a big show
As it should always to have been
Love overflowing
To all showing
That we love each other
One another
As sister and brother
Then in love we shall smother
All of the bad things
We will send them off by their wings
Then shall we have a love fling
Loving everything
For we shall be poised upon
love medicine.

New red shoes

Just in time
For a rhyme
About our love
From above
Just in time
For another rhyme
That the truth
Not be forsooth
Just in time
For a sign
That love is as strong
As love does live long
Just in time
For a little weeping
Love may be sad
Yet not ever bad
Just in time
For a little buying
New red shoes
Only for you
Just in time
For a little flying
All others ignored
Our love does soar
Just in time
For a little lying
A little sighing
A lot of trying.

LETTERS TO LEIGH

It is never too late

I love you and other than that
May I keep lesser words under my hat
Just as the sun does come up at dawn
My love shall arise to you then will fawn
Over you as the sun does the lawn
Then I will pledge to you my heart as a pawn
For it has been shown
Itself willing to be sawn
Into two halves
Waiting for your love salve
To make it whole again
Without my soul being in pain
Now here it is laying
Ready for your flaying
So goes the old saying
Along with my heart praying
That the path I am paving
Does lead toward my hearts craving
That I dreamt of last night
When inside of myself I had light
So that my love might
Grow bright
Without a fight
Or fit too tight
For as beside you I ever wait
It is never too late
To me you may escape
True love is never too late.

Take, hold, give

Take me to thy secret love
Hold me in thy hidden cove
Give loves craft a gentle shove
Take me to thy farthest shore
As we play on the sand
I will place a ring upon your hand
Then as we sit upon the land
We shall let our sea breeze be our fan.

LETTERS TO LEIGH

Your love is still proving

O father above heaven
Your love is still proving
That you endowed man
With part of your plan
A way of showing
The angels that have fallen
That an inferior human
Does not have to be like a demon
It is by choice
That we rebel or rejoice
In your law
As we have all saw
To be good
Just as we should
For what is to gain
From eternal pain
For that hellish fire
We have not a desire
Yet they call your way insane
Tho to us theirs is plain
For it is easy to see
That they are as insane as can be
Like the blind leading the blind
They cannot see what they have left behind
How could this world bring
Anything
Closer to being wise
Than those who seek paradise.

LETTERS TO LEIGH

For us he died

O holy father
May thy name be lauded
Forever and ever
Let thy name be hallowed
Myself should
Bear my wood
For it is a light load
With kind words to goad
Me on
To be one of thy earthly sons
To one day be to Jesus as a brother
For not another
May erase
Or replace
My soul that is stained
Forever cleansed by Jesus pain
For us he died
Cannot be denied
Then went he into the grave
Perhaps for the lost to save
On down into hell
then, if for him it were possible, to dispel
The sins of fallen angels
The first to evangel
Perhaps cleansing one such as myself of one
demon
Of those ways so heathen
He then rose on the third day
Showing to us the way.

LETTERS TO LEIGH

Through eternity

Let us laud
The name of the Lord
May
He receive the praise
Who can
Stand
In
His presence
The Lord Christ
Will be just
He shall cleanse
Us from sinful stains
From our flesh
Ugly pains
Only he does stand
To defend man
Against accusations
Of Satan's
Demons
Of whom
Will all kneel
In hell
The penalty
Through eternity
For bringing sin
To men
Then accursing them
He into following him.

LETTERS TO LEIGH

Now that you have taken all of our blame

O Jesus, do you still feel the same
Now that you have taken all of our blame
Is your pain less
The more that you are blessed
Or are you still sore
Where your flesh tore
When they hit you with whips
To have left that back in strips
Do you still
Feel
That you dwell
With thy holy grail
In reach
If we search
Then you may give
As we live
What we ever ask
For you that is a small task
Because your blood
By drops did flood
Then the saving ark
Was the fresh bark
That tore your shoulder
On your path toward the tombs boulder
Now your great door is open
By you hoping
That all will come in
So as to be freed of sin.

To save a remnant

Madness is in the air
Only Jesus stare
Does help to dispel
From hell
The influence of the angels
Who there-in fell
Who may tell
That it is a fiery well
Which those demons try to sell
As a pleasurable dell
Yet it is a cell
Waiting for the knell
Of judgement bells
All else pales
When fallen angels
Quell
Underneath their dark veil
Hearing each others wail
Turn into a yell
Yet be it with zeal
That I try to help
Anyone whose worth is as small as a nickel
By asking God please
We are all on our knees
Jesus was heaven sent
To save a remnant
Who for forever does repent.

LETTERS TO LEIGH

For one of his sheep

He will know
What
To do
To fix you
Where
Your
Spirit
Does need an extra merit
Do not be
Deceived
Before him
You cannot hide anything up your sleeve
Not by any slim
Chance
Not even if
In a trance
You offer up a gift
For he does own all
Even I heard his call
When
He came
For one of his sheep
Then you would learn to be meek
To turn the other cheek
A small price
Which the wise
Have found out
Does make the timid heart stout.

LETTERS TO LEIGH

Like an hourglass of sand

He does hold the desert in his hand
Like an hour glass of sand
Sparing a city for ten
Good men
That is a reason
To observe the season
That is warming
For a warning
That soon
The sun and moon
Will show portents
Moments
Before
The earth is tore
By a quake
As to prepare
For the lake
Of fire
For all
Who call
On Satan
To save them
Who does call them on
To have won
Their souls
With woes
Into hell
So does lead the tower of Babel and the devil.

LETTERS TO LEIGH

So long

I have been scarred
I have been scared
I know fear
I know that Jesus does care
Since he came
To take the blame
Of mans sin
Which does begin
When we are born
From earth torn
To appear on earth
Born of dirt
To bear
Our
Cross
Which is the cost
Of our lost
Paradise
Which does now lie
Underneath
Our feet
We may weep
In our sleep
We may cry
Then ask why
That it took so long, so long
For us to do wrong
While we failed to heed the angels song
For with Jesus we do belong.

LETTERS TO LEIGH

In thy book let mine be count

I love thee o father God
Tho I am made but out of sod
Back to dust I will return
After your love I do learn
That thy holy loving
Is being into me woven
That I then may
Find the way
Upward through the air
Up on the angels stairs
Please hold my hand
Up into the promised land
Please give me thy spiritual food
As I bear my cross of wood
I do not
Want
To let
You forget
That
I am just
A humble man
I do not know thy holy plan
I only play a minute
Part
Tho I am not astute
Nor am I smart
Yet if it is love that you want
In thy book let mine be count.

While the prophecy does unfold

Our souls
May bear the holes
From friendship
Then kins-lip
Speaking of love
Became a shove
When from above
Came a dove
Whose song
Made us to sing along
As our spirits then did rise
To guide through the lies
With other vice
the self-called wise
Of men
Full of sin
Continued
To elude
For they stayed unclean
Amidst the offered stream
Of living water
They would rather a slaughter
Before they confess
Jesus as blessed
Yet the story was told
In days of old
We just have to be bold
While the prophecy does unfold.

LETTERS TO LEIGH

Until the day

To silence the son
They would have to halt the father
Since that they cannot, they have begun
With the slaughter
Of innocent victims
Of this worlds system
An assault relentless
On those defenceless
Except for the saints call
That reaches
Gods kingdom hall
As Jesus teaches
Satan will fall
When from on high a call
Does say that this is the day God will
Do away
With Satan's evil
Into the pit he will be thrown
For his kingdom shall have fallen
No more will he trod
Upon the sod
Which was given
Life from heaven
What was heaven lent
Will return after it is spent
To the holy one
Who is with his holy son.

Then never let go

Jesus is calling men
He so does want to be our friend
If his goodness we accept
Then Satan's badness we reject
We sometimes do
Not know
What to
Do
When Satan on us does call
Yet we shall not fall
If we remember
That we are the Lords timber
Then to fell
Such
Jesus must touch
So as to heal
Our hearts
Within the inner parts
That were not quite whole
Like our souls
Because Satan
Took a part
Which he laid upon
His cart
Yet if we belong to Jesus
He will bless us
Then never let go
To always keep us from hells hole.

LETTERS TO LEIGH

May we love our brother

O Lord you are beautiful
Your way is so wonderful
For you took off your crown
Then came down
To earth
Where you humbled yourself to be born
Of dirt
Your glory shown
For a life span
A flash in the pan
In history
Quite a mystery
Would ourselves do the same
If we came
Down
To ease the frown
From lesser
Creatures
Is there one amongst
Us without faults
Whose life could pave
The way to save
May we love our brother
Enough to smother
Our feelings
With thoughts that are our self's killing
Let Jesus Christ be your brother
For unto man there is not another.

LETTERS TO LEIGH

To find the way

O Lord please heal my soul
That I may become whole
Allow myself to be a good servant
To help prevent
Foul sin
From sinking in
this body, I hope
your spirit will
Dwell
In and help me to cope
With my daily solutions
As I am breaking my resolutions
While I
Try
To find the way
Yet I must stay
Here
Where
Thee
Has placed me
In the gap
Of the map
Back from hell
Toward heavens bells
A lost sheep
Of which thee
Weep
While I just sleep.

LETTERS TO LEIGH

His gift

He came to end my strife
To bring to me life
Wanting for myself to have it in abundance
If I have not reluctance
To accept
His gift
So precious, life delicious
I hope then I pray
That he does not delay
To bring to me the words that pay
Another day
For what he says
Stays
Before me and through that I see
Hope
That I may cope
With a little faith
So that if I sayeth
Be thou removed, mountain
To uncover the living fountain
That is Christ
For we that thirst
Let us have love
Sent from above
For without love
Not anything in our treasure trove,
The Lords harp, scroll, and banner,
Having them without love I am yet a sinner.

LETTERS TO LEIGH

If we are bold

May I call you honey
Perhaps I will not be lonely
Please allow me to win
Then you may begin
To love me
As I love thee
You are bone of my bone
Even when we are not alone
You are flesh of my flesh
There I am caught in the mesh
Of your net
Yet
I cannot be caught
Because I have been bought
By heaven
Then to you given
So our love cannot be sold
If we are bold
Enough to take hold
Of this love
From above
That is heaven sent
To us lent
For our love we cannot repay
Tho let us say
That we may
Not be lonely
 if ever we are known as Robert and Leigh.

LETTERS TO LEIGH

The hand of Jesus

Everyone is in pain
On and off again
Something every week
That we all seek
To prolong
Beside of our song
That we sing
When life does bring
Something unpleasant
Then we are hesitant
To sing a sad song
For with love we do belong
We cannot go wrong
If we sing along
Tis the human condition
To live with some perdition
For we are made out of sod
Upon us the demons would trod
Yet back to dust we shall return
While in hell the demons will sojourn
Calling, Lord, please
Let our suffering ease
Then the pain will not cease
For then shall be too late that he should appease
So seize
The hand of Jesus
Your spirit will be at ease
Then your love will not cease.

This small town

All of the good people
Were looking up at the steeple
Where the Lords cross
Sheltered mans dross
All of the kind folk
Jabbed one another then did poke
Fun
At the one
Rejected stone
That the builders had shrunk from
For they had rated it
Unfit
For use
In doing so did refuse
The proper foundation
To build upon
Yet they cannot prevent
Judgement
From finding
Them and binding
Their evil
From the devil
Who is to be in hell
He shall there have fell
Dragging down
This small town
With a joke
Directed at these good folk.

LETTERS TO LEIGH

Then for love, heaven sent

Is love left
Am I to be bereft
For this love that I have felt
Some would have kilt
Then made me all alone
Yet you are still bone of my bone
My precious soap bubble
Ever my love puddle
That I would not bust
Even if I do thirst
To drink your dew
Always to drink you
Then touch your soul
That we may both become whole
I want you for my lady
Then to have my baby
We need to join
At hopes loin
Then let love begin
To hasten
Our sin
For being one another's friend
To the end
Then for love, heaven sent
To us lent
For we shall be one
Yet not alone
For our heart will have won.

With love and laughter

I cannot make it
Nor may I just sit
Here
With my tear
Falling down
Upon my frown
While
I wait on your smile
To shine
In a manner so fine
For my
Hearts eye
Then to stop the tear
That I within myself bear
For your memory
Is holding my heart stationary
As it is waiting
Anticipating
Our reunion
That will be so soothing
With love and laughter
After
We have kissed
Each other who we have missed
In love we shall be
Madly
Then love shall be adjusting
For our heart will be busting.

LETTERS TO LEIGH

My lonely one

I met a leprechaun
With hair light brown
She was full grown
A jewel in her crown
Within her pot
Was an ample lot
Of gold
All told
She was precious
More or less
With her own rainbow
For her lovers arrow
Which was in part
Imbedded in my heart
To pull it out
Would open my love fount
Then my blood of ruby
Would truly
Become a stream
In between
There would be my soul
Which is not quite whole
Because in my heart
Her lovers dart
Is in the part
Sent from heaven
My leprechaun,
 she is my lonely one.

No one else

My heart has been damaged
Yet my love has been salvaged
All of my love
From my hearts treasure trove
Does rest in your hand
Waiting to again make a plan
Of letting our love join
At loves loin
For love is to be reborn
The fleece of love is to be shorn
Which is my quest
To end in a love fest
Our love shall be reborn
Not to forever be forlorn
I love thee with a capital l
With our love we shall dispel
All of our fear
Along with each tear
Leaving to us bliss
Then such happiness
Within our home
As we are all alone
With ourselves
No one else
To cause us trouble
Or muddle
Up our love
Sent from above.

LETTERS TO LEIGH

To loosen loves coil

I do not
Want
You Leigh
To be
In the
Category
Of all
The rest
For you are the best
I only choose
You
To be
With me
Night and day
While I pray
That time
Will unwind
Then lead
Us to plead
To God
That he will give his nod
Saying then we
Be
Betrothed
As we let loves froth
Boil
Then may we toil
To loosen loves coil.

LETTERS TO LEIGH

I will adore

Her love is such
A touch
That does heal
When I so feel
Emotionally drained
Add to that heart felt pain
Her touch I miss
The touch of her kiss
May I forever remember
Her tender
Caress
For I confess
I trust
That my heart will not bust
Until
I feel
Her palm
Then hear her psalm
Again
While I plan
Never
To sever
Ever
Forever
More
I will adore
My little dove,
Such a, o my, treasure trove.

LETTERS TO LEIGH

The love of two

How long must I call
On my love
Shall I far fall
Little dove
How long must I wait
To learn loves fate
How tall
Shall
The love of two
Grow
When shall we learn
That love does not ever burn
Without leaving a tender scar
Soon after placing a bar
Across that place
Such a special space
Inside
Of my heart
Beside
That part
Where the pain
Shall cease
When again
I will ease
Into loves pool
Then be loves fool.

The love that I borrow

Come tomorrow
I will have not fear
To swallow
Only a tear
Here
Even there
In the hollow
Of my heart
In that part
Where the love that I borrow
Shall grow
Then show
Fruit
Of truth
For our
Love
Shall
Not fall
While
Like others
Guile
They separate
That holy state
Of marriage for some
Reason
Or another
Yet one shall the other be healing
Always with that loving feeling.

LETTERS TO LEIGH

With Jesus Christ

Let us place
Our trust in the Lord
May he be our mace
May his sword
Be
Before
Around and after
Then may we have laughter
For we are in his arms
Safe from harm
From all alarm
For with him we are calm
In the face of the storm
Which into this world we are born
Not to be alone
Only to sing along
With others
Our brothers
In this life
Of less strife
With Jesus Christ
Who is the first
Our Lord
The saviour
Who lives above
From where he does give
To us love.

LETTERS TO LEIGH

Tender feelings

Again
I begin
To let
My eyes grow wet
Over my loss
Yet the cross
Is light
For then my eyes grow bright
When you I see
Looking at me
Across space
I see your face
That is when I begin
Again
To count
What I had fount
As blessed
Not distressed
Like some
For I hope to have won
Your love so fair
Yes, and pleasantly square
For being with you night and day
Always
Does put me in touch
With such
A tender feeling
Of that emotional healing.

LETTERS TO LEIGH

I shall find out tomorrow

I love you lady
I love you today
I love all of your being
That I am seeing
I do not call you by your name
For I am not ready to add to your fame
Yet I see you every Sunday
With your platter and your tray
Take my heart upon your platter
For to me it does not matter
Lay my love upon your tray
Then with your own let it play
O beautiful woman
O your beauty can
Stir my heart
Tho we are apart
Your beauty for my lonely eye
Does make my love fly
Are there words enough
To describe your beautiful touch
As for your voice
Hush all noise
So that I may hear
What has not a peer
O beautiful eyes
Full of sighs
I shall find out tomorrow
If me they do follow.

LETTERS TO LEIGH

We shall our love mix

I am sitting in my corner
Of my love I am a mourner
Yet I do not hate
Because we may resuscitate
All of this tender feeling
That may lead to a healing
Of our emotion
For we shall come to a solution
There will be not any bitter pollution
When we make our love potion
Because when you are Mrs. Nix
We shall our love mix
Together
Into a better
Brew
From which we shall drink
As we into love sink
Then if we
Need
A refill
We shall stand and fulfil
Anew
The fire
That we shall stir
As the sparks do fly
High
Into the sky
Then there will not be more good-byes.

LETTERS TO LEIGH

Be at ease

Please
Let my heart
Be at ease
Then let it start
To
Overflow
With thy love
From above
To let thy grace
Shine into my face
From day to day
That I may
Say
Hallowed is thy name
Mighty be thy fame
Strong is thy arm
That does keep us from harm
Night and day
In ever way
Hold us in thy glove
To keep us in thy love
May thy love ease
May we thou please
With our prayers
That are forever
On our lips
While on thy love we sip.

LETTERS TO LEIGH

Begging you to bring your tear

Someday I hope for you to read this
I hope for you to feel some soothing bliss
Knowing that I love you so
Then continued to woo
While you were far away
To where you so long had to stay
Yet if you are reading this it is known
That from that place you may have flown
You will have found me with open arms
To escape the following storms
You always knew that I was here
Begging you to bring your tear
I knew how to end your fear
For you began a new life when you left your bier
I have saved some money
To help you feel like a honey
You just may have fled
Into my bed
Leaving the strife
To become my wife
For unto you I will not say no
Oh God, let it be so
You are all that I want in life
I shall truly love you as my wife
Let me forever love you please
I am already on my knees
Please come soon
I hope by noon.

LETTERS TO LEIGH

Who can come

Though I am in a place of shame
We will soon hear of my fame
If anyone is out there
Who may straighten my affair
Please do not hesitate
Please do not be too late
To come out on this limb
Then tenderly help to ease my mind
For forever will I call you friend.

LETTERS TO LEIGH

I thank God

O Lord, I am just a sinner
To do your will I am ever a beginner
Please give to me thy spiritual food
To help me through my moods
For man does not live by bread alone
Only to have the holy spirit in his bones
Is a spiritual compass
To avoid a satanic impasse
Where many have there-in fell
On into the gaping jaws of hell
For the devil
Is everywhere
Spreading evil
Here and there
Laying traps for men
To tempt them into sin
Because it is his fashion
To devour us with a passion
So let us be on guard
For some that may be hard
I thank God
That I am made of sod
For back to dust I will return
While my spirit does churn
On an upward climb
While I am sure to find
That I left behind
The troubles of my mind.

LETTERS TO LEIGH

Never leaving you behind

Love is a tender trap
Like a plant whose sap
Rises then falls
With echoes and then calls
Me on
To find where love does come from
Looking for that
Tender trap
As I go about
The day without
Your face
Yet it is in a safe place,
A special space
With my hearts pace
Beating along
With your song
Inside of my mind
Never leaving you behind
You are always with me
Through your vision I see
The world a-new
With skies of blue
Then pearly clouds
Bestow a bow
While pouring down
Upon our frown
Love, that tender trap
Whose sap we hope to tap.

LETTERS TO LEIGH

If you would only wear my ring

I am living like a king
Custom smokes and everything
Yet my good fortune does not bring
You to me for you to sing
While my heart mends
I have made new friends
Tho you they cannot erase
You they cannot replace
I am making progress in my health
Steadily growing in wealth
To you I would give everything
If you would only wear my ring
I have new clothes
I have new shoes
I have new holes
In my heart and soul
That only you may fill
Which only I can feel
You I shall never replace
For in my heart will always be a trace
Of your taste
That I will never waste
Baby, you are not to blame
Yet it is a shame
That a love like ours
Should ever grow sour
That is why I still let
My face grow wet.

LETTERS TO LEIGH

I just cannot believe

If you wonder why I do write in red
These are the drops that my heart has bled
These are the tears that my soul has shed
This is the life that I have led
Since you have went away
With another life to play
I did not want it to be that way
Yet dues of life we must pay
I guess that I am doing alright
For everywhere you are in my sight
Then I rise and turn on the light
I do not look for pleasure from my toys
You know how it is with boys
I have almost lost all of my poise
Here no one may say that he ever enjoys,
I have your picture that is true
Tho I am not able to hold that like I did you
I am ill and turning blue
Maybe I have the love flu
I just cannot believe
That anyone is able to love you as much as me
Only this you may relieve
If you again refer to us as we
I will squeeze out a bit more blood
That is I would,
I could,
I should.

LETTERS TO LEIGH

Within your hidden cove

Only another day
For love to come and play
Just another way
For me to say
Of you I do think
Of you I then blink
Back the tear
That the fear
Of losing you
May come true
I am thinking sure
My love is not poor
It may handle
Loves short candle
All will not melt
Until you have felt
My simple love
Within your hidden cove
Take me there-in
As a friend
Hold me close
Then do not lose
My love that you have found
With which you are bound
To take care of
Like a mourning dove
Over her fallen mate
Give to me love not too late.

LETTERS TO LEIGH

She does not even wonder why

We came from kings
Now all that I have is a silver ring
We once owned slaves
Yet now they share my cave
I am just white trash
Without land, little cash
The landlord is knocking at the door
There is not enough chairs, we sit on the floor
Mama is working like a fool
We all act up at school
When it is our turn to do the dishes
We just sat there making wishes
If it is time to make the beds
We walk by and shake our heads
Mama pulls up on the pave
We are putting her in an early grave
She is too tired to clean the house
Or to worry if we have a mouse
She will get to that tomorrow
If she makes it through today's sorrow
Then we all get into a line
Just in time to whine
Mama hands out the last few cents
Of the work money that she has been lent
Never to complain, nor to cry
She does not even wonder why
Only does she wish that there was more to bring
Home to the kids that came from kings.

Trembling lips

Trembling lips tell me why
Trembling lips please do not lie
In my dreams you still slip by
Over you my heart does yet sigh
It has been some days then some years
Some weeping then some tears
Never seeing you is my fear
With me you have not a peer
I wake up yet stay
Laid down
With my frown
Then I review
My dreams
Anew
For I so hope that you are in the scenes
If I
Do not find
You
I may shed a tear or two
In my heart
Where my love did start
That day
I heard you say
I am bone of your bone
Even
When
We are both alone.

LETTERS TO LEIGH

To a better place

All of the gold under Egypt
Is not legit
For someone to buy
The look in my eye
When you I often see
Looking at me
All of the wealth of Babylon
Is not worth looking upon
When I have you as a light
Within my sight
All of this besides
The lost ten tribes
Cannot ransom
My love from your person
My love for you I cannot stop
This love for you I cannot top
You set me to spinning
Then leave me grinning
In my mouth your taste
I shall not waste
I would love to go out with your love and play
To forever play day after day
After that, if ever we came in
We should dance and dance again
Until we grew tired
Then wished to retire
To a better place
Then there unlace.

LETTERS TO LEIGH

Before you travel

Ever since I first met you
I thought you worthy of a poem or two
Perhaps more
Maybe I will not bore
Yet you are the type that I have been looking for
Dark of hair and creamier of pore
If this you softly ignore
I will softly still adore
Allow me three months time
I shall put a three-hundred page book on line
Dedicated to your beauty
As a poet it is my duty
To find the fairest flower
Which does not always tower
Above the others
Yet does sit quietly with one another
Saving their fair nod
For their passing God
Will I therefore not say
Without delay
That you have something that I call class
I hope your heart is not of brass
For if there was something here to do
I would find a way to woo
As I hope to unravel
Before you travel
Your hearts strings
 I may with them yet sing.

LETTERS TO LEIGH

Yet my favourite is of love

These are just odd poems
You have not arrived to the good ones
They are locked up inside of my secret place
Covered by precious feathers and delicate lace
This one is floating out now
Uncovering another somehow
I do not know how many more
Are closer to the floor
Tho the one coming is at the top
For that whatever I do cannot it stop
The man inside of me is a natural poet
When I feel beauty I do not like to stow it
Behind being macho
Because I am not in that way mucho
Of that I tell you not a lie
I may write poems that could bring tears to the eye
Followed with what would make you giggle
Then laugh and cough and wiggle
I should write about God
That you may solemnly nod
Or about nature
Of observing her rapture
Yet my favourite is of love
Who sometimes does need a little shove
To help her get her job done
Then we would not all be alone
All of this has come from Pandora's box
While she has lost her locks.

LETTERS TO LEIGH

As certain as the dew

I will be there for you
Children and baby too
I will be there for you
When the skies are darkest blue
I will be there for you
When all of the others are through
I will be there for you
When you do not have a clue
I will be there for you
With holes in my shoe
I will be there for you
Wondering what to do
I will be there for you
(all the time you knew)
I will be there for you
With teardrops not a few
I will be there for you
As if just on cue
I will be there for you
As certain as the dew
I will be there for you
Just like a lost Jew
I will be there for you
Not sitting in my pew
I will be there for you
So go ahead and sue.

LETTERS TO LEIGH

Leigh's dilemma

I am doing
Time
While I am wooing
In my mind
I have done wrong things
Now my punishment may end
For now I sing
With the love that you send
Yet why
Did you go out for
Beer
When I have champagne
At home
Are not my thighs as silky
Is not my skin as milky
Are not my breast
As pleasant
Is not my hair
As fair
Are not my lips
Gentle whips
That drive me on
Bone of your bone
Flesh of your flesh
Champagne taste
On my tongue baste
So why leave me for her
For just a beer,

LETTERS TO LEIGH

Leigh's dilemma cont.

Now I am just sitting here
Waiting for my tear
To fall
Yet that is not all
You have left me
Now I see
Why you go out for beer
When you have champagne right here
You go out alone
When you have champagne at home
Why do you rove
When you have my love
To keep you home
Yet I am alone
Again
Alone with my champagne
Why go out for beer
When you have my pure
Tears
That sear
Their way
Into my heart to stay
As you roam around
Town
For something to drink
While into tears I have sank
So why go out for beer
When you have champagne right here.

LETTERS TO LEIGH

And know

I do not
Want
You to think that my love is not clean
Nor to think that my love is mean
I may have said some dirty words
Yet I do not take for granted your sheath and my
sword
I will love you forever and ever
No other girl will ever sever
The friendship that we have
That I will always save
Our love grew little by little
As I sought to solve that loving riddle
About what I thought if you could have a black
child
As I write I have solved the riddle and know that it
is now fulfilled
I am telling you that I would not have minded
For we have five left that are likewise mix-skinned
I shall love you through thick and thin
Then your love I shall finally win
In that day we will be bold
As our story will finally be told
Your heart, your heart, your heart I love
Yes, my love for you I will ever prove
For we shall finally one day meet
How will my heart you then treat
Shall depend on if for me your love does yet glow
For even
In
The dark

LETTERS TO LEIGH

My love will hark
And know.

Loving is not a sin

Some of my friends seem to be
Turning on me
Yet I hope that you never will be,
Leigh
I believe
That you will always
See
Me
As a friend
With a heart to lend
With love to send
So your own may mend
Because
I love you without pause
On through the years
With the lonely tears
Then the fears
That through my mind sear
I hope on knowing that without faith
I cannot sayeth
That we will meet again
For being faithless is kind of like a sin
In
That state I do not want to be
I would like for my faith to be free
 until you see
Me
Again
Loving is not a sin.

LETTERS TO LEIGH

Love

Leigh,
How am I say
Good-bye
To thee
I waited
My heart waited
For thee
For over ten years
For ten years my heart and soul did bleed
Love
Is forgetting good enough
For me forgetting is pretty tough
You said that you would see me
In eternity
How may that not be enough
For then our hearts may forever touch
My soul continued to
My heart continued to
Love brew
I cannot allow
Myself to love
As much love
As I possess
For I
Often love
Others
More
Than
My self
Yet
I love.

LETTERS TO LEIGH

The end,
Yet perhaps, not.

www.ingramcontent.com/pod-product-compliance
Lightning Source LLC
Chambersburg PA
CBHW020653270326
41928CB00005B/101

* 9 7 8 1 8 4 7 4 7 3 9 9 8 *